Barbara O'Neill's
Lost and Forgotten Apothecary Revived

Copyright © 2024 by Margaret Willowbrook

All rights reserved. No part of this publication may be reproduced, distributed, or transmitted in any form or by any means, including photocopying, recording, or other electronic or mechanical methods, without the prior written permission of the publisher, except in the case of brief quotations embodied in critical reviews and certain other noncommercial uses permitted by U.S. copyright law. For permission requests, write to the publisher at the address below.

A Better You Everyday Publications
Email: info@abetteryoueveryday.com

Disclaimer
The information provided in this book is for educational and informational purposes only and is not affiliated with, authorized, endorsed by, or in any way officially connected with Barbara O'Neill or her affiliates or subsidiaries. The use of Barbara O'Neill's name in this book is for explanatory, educational, and reference purposes only, to discuss and provide insight into the theories and practices she has publicized through her teachings and public appearances. The views and interpretations presented in this book solely reflect those of the author and have not been reviewed or approved by Barbara O'Neill or her representatives.

The content within this book is not intended as medical advice and should not be taken as such. The author, Margaret Willowbrook, is not a medical professional. This book should not replace consultation with a qualified healthcare professional. It is essential that before beginning any new health practice, you consult with your physician, especially if you have any pre-existing health conditions.

While every effort has been made to verify the information provided in this book, the field of natural health is dynamic, and as such, the content may not reflect the most recent research or medical consensus. The author and publisher assume no responsibility for errors, omissions, or contrary interpretations of the subject matter herein.

Readers are encouraged to confirm the information contained within this publication through independent research and professional advice. Any perceived slights of specific people or organizations are unintentional. By reading this book, you agree that the author and publisher are not responsible for the success or failure of your health decisions related to any information presented.

A Better You Everyday Publications
email address info@abetteryoueveryday.com

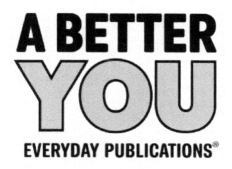

www.abetteryoueveryday.com

Barbara O'Neill's Lost and Forgotten Apothecary Revived

250 Ancient Remedies for Modern Wellness

By Margaret Willowbrook

USA
2024

TABLE OF CONTENTS

GLIMPSE INTO THE CHAPTERS AHEAD. 1

FOREWORD. 7

INTRODUCTION. 9

    How to Use This Book. 10

    The Legacy of Barbara O'Neill 11

PART I: FOUNDATIONS OF A HOME APOTHECARY. 13

CHAPTER 1: EQUIPPING YOUR APOTHECARY (TOOLS, ESSENTIAL EQUIPMENT, STORAGE SOLUTIONS) 15

    The Legacy of Barbara O'Neill 15

PART I: FOUNDATIONS OF A HOME APOTHECARY 19

CHAPTER 1: EQUIPPING YOUR APOTHECARY (TOOLS, ESSENTIAL EQUIPMENT, STORAGE SOLUTIONS) 21

CHAPTER 2: SOURCING AND IDENTIFYING HERBS (FORAGING BASICS, ETHICAL HARVESTING, REPUTABLE SUPPLIERS, GROWING YOUR OWN) 23

CHAPTER 3: PREPARATION TECHNIQUES (INFUSIONS, DECOCTIONS, TINCTURES, OILS, VINEGARS, SYRUPS, SALVES, POULTICES, OXYMELS, PROPER DOSAGE) 27

PART II: REMEDIES FOR COMMON AILMENTS. 31

CHAPTER 4: DIGESTIVE HEALTH AND METABOLISM (REMEDIES 1–40) 33

CHAPTER 5: RESPIRATORY AND IMMUNE SUPPORT (REMEDIES 41–80) 49

CHAPTER 6: SKIN AND HAIR CARE (REMEDIES 81–110) 65

CHAPTER 7: STRESS, MOOD, AND SLEEP AIDS (REMEDIES 111–140) 77

CHAPTER 8: WOMEN'S WELLNESS AND FAMILY HEALTH (REMEDIES 141–170) 89

CHAPTER 9: JOINT, MUSCLE, AND MOBILITY SUPPORT (REMEDIES 171–200) 101

CHAPTER 10: ENERGY AND VITALITY (REMEDIES 201–220) . 113

CHAPTER 11: SEASONAL TONICS AND YEAR-ROUND WELLBEING (REMEDIES 221–235) 121

CHAPTER 12: KITCHEN APOTHECARY (REMEDIES 236–245) . 127

CHAPTER 13: CULTURAL AND TRADITIONAL REMEDIES (REMEDIES 246–250) 133

CHAPTER 14: SAFETY GUIDELINES AND WHEN TO SEEK PROFESSIONAL ADVICE (CONTRAINDICATIONS, PEDIATRIC USE, PREGNANCY PRECAUTIONS, MEDICATION INTERACTIONS) 137

CHAPTER 15: PRESERVING KNOWLEDGE AND PASSING IT FORWARD (KEEPING AN HERBAL JOURNAL, SHARING WISDOM, FURTHER READING AND RESOURCES) 145

CONCLUSION. 155

LAST WORD. 157

GLOSSARY OF HERBAL TERMS 159

CONVERSION TABLES. 163

REFERENCES 165

BONUS PAGE: VIDEO SHORT TUTORIALS BY BARBARA O'NEILL 167

GLIMPSE INTO THE CHAPTERS AHEAD.

As you begin your journey through these pages, it may be helpful to know what lies ahead and how each chapter is designed to guide you. Together, they form a tapestry of herbal wisdom that blends time-honored traditions with modern needs, giving you both the understanding and the practical skills to incorporate natural remedies into your daily life. Think of this overview as a map that will help you navigate from basic knowledge to specific topics, ultimately encouraging you to embrace a more harmonious relationship with nature's pharmacy.

In the early chapters, you will lay the foundation that will support your entire practice.

Chapter 1: Equipping Your Apothecary introduces the essential tools, containers, and organizational strategies that will set you up for success and ensure that you always have what you need close at hand.

Chapter 2: Sourcing and Identifying Herbs teaches you where to find quality plant material, whether you are foraging in the wild, purchasing from reputable suppliers, or growing your own. You will learn how to distinguish beneficial herbs from look-alikes, and discover the importance of ethical harvesting and sustainable practices.

Chapter 3: Preparation Techniques then reveals the methods for transforming raw plant parts into effective remedies. From simple infusions and decoctions to tinctures, ointments, and syrups, these instructions empower you to unlock the healing potential of every herb. With this strong foundation, you will be ready to explore remedies designed for specific purposes.

Chapter 4: Digestive Health and Metabolism delves into herbs that calm the stomach, support nutrient absorption, and promote overall digestive balance. These preparations can help address everyday discomfort, promote regularity, and maintain a resilient gut environment. Moving on,

Chapter 5: Respiratory and Immune Support focuses on remedies to clear congestion, relieve coughs, support lung function, and strengthen your body's defenses. Whether you are facing seasonal challenges or seeking long-term resilience, this section offers practical solutions inspired by herbal traditions.

Chapter 6: Skin and Hair Care shifts the focus outward, exploring preparations that restore skin's natural radiance and add vitality and strength to your hair. From gentle cleansers to nourishing oils and conditioners, you will find ways to enhance your appearance while maintaining the integrity of your body's protective barrier.

Chapter 7: Aids for Stress, Mood, and Sleep recognizes the profound connection between emotional well-being and physical health. Here you will discover herbs that calm anxious minds, promote restful sleep, and uplift the spirit, offering a gentle path to inner balance.

Chapter 8: Women's Wellness and Family Health addresses the unique needs of women and families at different stages of life. You will learn about ways to ease menstrual cramps, support healthy lactation, soothe children's minor ailments, and navigate the transitions of menopause with confidence and grace.

Chapter 9: Joint, Muscle, and Mobility Support turns attention to the body's structural foundation. By exploring herbs and techniques that relieve pain, improve circulation, and maintain flexibility, this section provides tools for staying active and comfortable as you move through the demands of daily life.

Chapter 10: Energy and Vitality focuses on building and maintaining natural strength, alertness, and endurance over time. Rather than relying on quick fixes, you will learn about remedies that nourish and energize the body from the inside out, laying the groundwork for lasting stamina.

Chapter 11: Seasonal Tonics and Year-Round Well-Being encourages you to align your health practices with the rhythms of nature. By adapting your herbal choices to the changing seasons, you can harmonize with the cycles of growth, harvest, and rest that shape both the plant world and your own inner balance.

In Chapter 12, The Kitchen Pharmacy, you will discover that some of the best remedies may already be waiting in your pantry. Everyday spices, fruits, and culinary herbs can be transformed into powerful allies, proving that nature's pharmacy is often closer than we think.

Chapter 13: Cultural and Traditional Remedies broadens your perspective and connects you to traditions from around the world. By exploring healing practices passed down through generations and across continents, you will appreciate the universal human quest for wellness and the diverse ways people have partnered with plants to achieve it.

Chapter 14: Safety Guidelines and When to Seek Professional Advice provides a framework for recognizing potential contraindications, understanding dosage and preparation limits, and knowing when to consult health care providers. This chapter empowers you to incorporate natural remedies into your life with caution and integrity, safeguarding your well-being and that of your loved ones.

Finally, Chapter 15: Preserving and Passing on Knowledge encourages you to become a steward of this legacy. By keeping records, sharing insights, and continuing to learn, you can help preserve these traditions for future generations. You will find suggestions for further reading, ways to deepen your education, and methods to ensure that the wisdom you have gained remains alive, relevant, and accessible.

At the end of the book, the Glossary of Herbal Terms clarifies specialized vocabulary, and conversion tables ensure accurate measurements for consistent results. These resources support everything you learn, making your herbal explorations more efficient, informed, and rewarding.

Taken together, these chapters provide a comprehensive journey. You will move from setting up your apothecary to addressing specific health concerns, from understanding time-honored cultural traditions to ensuring safety and continuity of knowledge. Along the way, you will gain the skills and confidence to integrate nature's remedies into your daily routine. This book aims not only to inform and educate, but also to inspire a lasting connection with the plants that have long provided comfort, nourishment, and healing. May this journey help you find your own path in the ever-evolving world of herbal wisdom.

Attention!

Before you get into this captivating book, we have an exclusive offer just for you! A fantastic FREE Bonus:

Get Your Ready-to-Print Herbal Reference Guide Bonuses!

Remedy Recipes (6 pages) — EXPLORE A VARIETY OF NATURAL, EASY-TO-PREPARE REMEDY RECIPES FOR DAILY HEALTH NEEDS, SPANNING STRESS RELIEF TO IMMUNE SUPPORT.

Herbal First Aid (4 pages) — ACCESS DETAILED HERBAL SOLUTIONS FOR COMMON HEALTH ISSUES, PROVIDING NATURAL EMERGENCY CARE ALTERNATIVES.

Herb Directory (6 pages) — DELVE INTO AN EXTENSIVE DIRECTORY OF MEDICINAL HERBS, COMPLETE WITH USES, BENEFITS, AND PREPARATION TIPS.

These printable guides, crafted after extensive research and dedication, offer quick, easy access to a wealth of herbal remedies, recipes, and first aid information. Designed for fast reference, they cover everything from specific herbs in our 'Herb Directory', to swift recipes in 'Remedy Recipes', and practical emergency care in 'Herbal First Aid'. Though we plan to sell them separately in the future, we're currently offering these guides for free as our appreciation for your book purchase, as a way of saying thank you and adding extra value to your reading experience.

For instant delivery, simply chat with our Facebook bot via the link below or scan the accompanying QR code.

http://tinyurl.com/Herbalbonuses

Alternatively, you can request the guides by emailing us at: info@abetteryoueveryday.com.
Enjoy your reading and these additional resources!

Foreword.

When I first came across the old notebook bearing Barbara O'Neill's name, it was tucked away in a dusty corner of an attic, its pages curled and yellowed by time. There was something about the careful handwriting and faded ink drawings that spoke of a life of patience, observation, and respect for the quiet gifts of nature. I remember feeling as if I had opened a window into another era, one in which herbal traditions were not only known, but lived and breathed every day. As I studied these pages, I saw more than leaves and roots. I saw a tapestry of centuries of wisdom passed down through whispers and loving hands. These remedies were more than instructions; they were stories, and in each infusion, salve, or tonic, I could hear voices sharing knowledge over kitchen tables as herbs gently dried above. The remedies that now fill this book are drawn from that legacy, distilled into a guide you can hold in your hands. Here you will find teas to soothe an upset stomach, potions to calm the mind, salves to soothe the body, and elixirs to warm the soul. Each one forms a bond that connects you to the generations who have turned to nature for comfort and healing. My hope is that you will find something here that resonates with you, something that helps you find comfort, courage, or renewed vitality in your own life. It is an honor to bring these forgotten treasures into the present, to pay tribute to Barbara O'Neill, and to place this key to ancient wisdom in your hands. May you carry it forward and make these ancient gifts blossom again.

Margaret Willowbrook

Introduction.

At the heart of this collection is a simple and enduring truth: nature has always held the potential to guide us toward wellness and balance. These remedies, drawn from the forgotten apothecary of Barbara O'Neill and lovingly gathered here, invite us to reconnect with traditions that transcend time. Each recipe is a small window into a world where careful observation and respect for the earth's bounty can help us find harmony within.

For this introduction, consider the serene landscapes and gentle rhythms that surround us. Imagine the rolling fields of wildflowers, the forest floor softly carpeted with moss, the clear streams and their whispering currents. In these places grows the raw material for the tonics, teas, infusions, and tinctures that fill these pages. Many of these remedies have been almost lost to memory, overshadowed by the fast pace and convenience of modern life. Yet here they are, waiting patiently to restore what has been put aside.

As you read, remember that each remedy is more than a means to relieve discomfort. It is a reminder of the partnership we can forge with the living world. It encourages us to step beyond the pharmacy aisle and trust in the generosity of nature. In turning to these recipes, we welcome a slow return to wisdom and a thoughtful embrace of the ingredients that have soothed countless generations before us.

Let these pages be your companion. They are not a substitute for medical advice or professional care, but rather a gentle nudge toward wholeness. May they fill your pantry with fragrant herbs and healing roots, your kitchen with the aroma of simmering brews, and your daily life with small acts of nourishment. May these recipes plant a seed in your mind and heart, helping you to remember that old ways can still hold new promise.

Margaret Willowbrook

How to Use This Book.

This book has been created as both a guide and a companion to help you weave the gifts of nature into your daily life. Whether you are new to herbal traditions or have relied on them for a long time, you will find here a carefully structured collection designed to lead you step by step into the world of ancient remedies and practical preparations.

Start by reading the basic chapters. They will give you insight into equipping your apothecary, sourcing ingredients responsibly, and mastering basic techniques. Once you are familiar with these basics, approach the remedies with an open mind and a spirit of curiosity. Each recipe includes a name, a brief description of its intended use, and instructions for preparation. The ingredients are natural and often readily available, and the instructions are meant to be followed with care and reverence.

Move through the chapters as your interests and needs guide you. If you are drawn to digestive health, explore the section dedicated to easing stomach discomfort. If restful sleep is elusive, explore the soothing blends that have soothed many before you. Keep this book handy in your kitchen or next to your favorite reading chair, and refer to it when life's inevitable discomforts arise.

To take full advantage of these remedies, gather fresh or high-quality dried herbs, invest time in understanding their properties, and treat each preparation as an opportunity to connect with the rhythms of nature. Along the way, use the glossary and charts in the appendices for additional reference, and consider taking notes on your own experiences. Adjust recipes slightly if you find they work better that way, and note which herbs and preparations bring you comfort. In doing so, you become part of a lineage that stretches back through countless generations who have found balance and well-being in the healing gifts of the earth.

THE LEGACY OF BARBARA O'NEILL.

In the quiet corners of old homesteads and hidden gardens, Barbara O'Neill once walked with unwavering curiosity, seeking the gentle remedies that had guided countless lives before her. She was not famous in her time, not a household name or a celebrated figure in history. Instead, her reputation was quietly spread by word of mouth, recognized by neighbors, friends, and those who understood that true healing is often found in the most unlikely places. These pages you now hold trace their lineage back to her careful notes, recorded in small journals that smelled of pressed flowers and dried leaves. As she accumulated knowledge over decades, Barbara O'Neill developed a deep intimacy with her surroundings. She learned the language of leaves, the whispers of blossoms, and the soft hum of roots burrowing into rich soil. What came from her pen was neither formula nor doctrine, but guidance. Her remedies were never imposed, and each was chosen with respect for its source. Just as a loved one might share a favorite family recipe, she wrote as if sharing a treasured secret, encouraging readers to remain humble stewards of the earth's gifts. Through these lessons, Barbara O'Neill demonstrated that wellness is not a final destination, but a lifelong journey. We now stand at a crossroads where modern convenience meets ancient wisdom. By opening this book and welcoming her guidance into your life, you will help ensure that her legacy continues to flourish in the gardens of the future.

Part I: Foundations of a Home Apothecary.

Before you dive into the world of natural remedies, it is wise to lay a solid foundation. The chapters in this section will introduce you to the tools and techniques needed to create herbal concoctions that support wellness. By learning how to properly equip your apothecary, source and identify the herbs you need, and master basic preparation methods, you will build the skills and confidence necessary to explore the full range of remedies that follow. Think of this section as the sturdy roots beneath a thriving garden, providing nourishment and structure so that the leaves and flowers above can flourish.

Chapter 1: Equipping Your Apothecary (Tools, Essential Equipment, Storage Solutions).

A well-equipped apothecary is like a reliable kitchen, stocked with utensils and staples that make any recipe easy to try. Whether you plan to make a simple herbal tea or a more elaborate tincture, having the right tools can make all the difference. Start with the basics: clean glass jars and bottles, strainers, a mortar and pestle for crushing herbs, and an assortment of spoons and measuring cups. A good pair of scissors and a sharp knife will help you cut roots and leaves. Muslin or cheesecloth can be used to sieve out small particles, while funnels help prevent spills. Once you have gathered your equipment, consider how best to store your herbs. Keep them in a cool, dry place out of direct sunlight. Label jars clearly with the name of the herb and the date you collected or purchased it. Over time, you will learn to maintain a pantry filled with nature's treasures, each shelf supporting your journey into herbal practice. By ensuring that your workspace is both organized and inviting, you set the stage for success. Soon you will be exploring the essential knowledge needed to identify, source, and prepare your herbs with confidence and care.

The Legacy of Barbara O'Neill

To understand the true depth and meaning of these remedies, it is helpful to first appreciate the legacy of Barbara O'Neill. Although the records of her life are sparse, often passed down through oral histories and personal diaries, we know enough to piece together a portrait of a remarkable herbalist who wove practicality, compassion, and a deep respect for nature into her work. She was not a famous physician, nor did she boast extensive academic credentials, but what she did possess was an unwavering belief in the healing power of the plants around her.

Barbara lived in a time when many families relied on what grew in their backyards and along country roads. Through seasons of scarcity and abundance, people turned to her for guidance. She studied the habits of wild herbs, learned the best times to harvest, and understood how to preserve the beneficial properties of roots, leaves, and flowers. She knew to wait for the early morning dew to gather herbs at their most potent, and to hang them carefully in a cool, dry place so that their flavors and healing properties would not be lost. She understood that wellness was more than just treating symptoms. It was a balance achieved by attending to the body, mind, and spirit alike.

In her small journals, she noted the best ways to soothe a crying infant with a gentle chamomile infusion or to ease a laboring mother's discomfort with a raspberry leaf tonic. She offered advice to neighbors suffering from persistent coughs or lingering fevers, often incorporating accessible local plants into simple recipes. Her approach was patient and observant. She watched her remedies in action, noting subtle changes in color, aroma, and effect. Over time, she honed her practice, refining and improving her formulas. In this way, her knowledge deepened and her reputation grew.

The importance of Barbara O'Neill's legacy lies not only in the remedies themselves, but in the perspective they promote. They remind us that wellness is accessible without the need for complex machinery or expensive ingredients. They invite us to slow down and examine the qualities of the plants that grow around us. They suggest that a well-stocked home apothecary can be more than a repository of remedies. It can be a testament to our enduring connection to the living world. By learning from her legacy, we bring these ancient traditions forward, not as relics of the past, but as practical solutions to modern challenges.

In studying Barbara's methods, we can take note of her patient observation and willingness to adapt. Her work shows that our ancestors were not just passive recipients of nature's bounty. They were active participants in the subtle dance between plants and humans. This relationship thrives when we recognize that every cup of tea, every soothing balm, and every simple infusion is more than a quick fix. It is an opportunity to nourish ourselves and strengthen our connection to the natural world.

As you continue to explore the remedies in this book, remember that they are part of this heritage. These traditions can be embraced by anyone who is willing to learn to identify local resources and show respect for the plants themselves. As you sip a fragrant infusion or apply a gentle ointment, remember that you are not only tending to your immediate needs. You are also carrying forward a candle of knowledge lit by those who came before us. In doing so, you will ensure that Barbara O'Neill's legacy remains alive and accessible for generations to come.

Part I: Foundations of a Home Apothecary

Before you start mixing tonics or measuring out precise spoonfuls of dried flowers and roots, it is important to understand the basic principles and tools that will support your journey. A well-prepared home apothecary serves as both a workshop and a sanctuary. It contains the tools that allow you to transform raw plant materials into healing preparations. It contains the references and notes that guide your choices. Most importantly, it provides a dedicated space for thoughtful and informed herbal work.

Think of this basic section as your guide to setting the stage. You will discover what tools are essential, what ingredients to have on hand, and how best to store them. You will learn how to identify plants and find reliable sources for herbs. You will become familiar with the primary techniques used to extract the valuable qualities of each plant, whether by steeping them in hot water, blending them into oils, or reducing them into syrups.

These chapters provide the core knowledge that will allow you to approach the rest of the book with confidence. Without a solid foundation, the most advanced remedies can feel overwhelming or fail to deliver their potential benefits. By starting here, you will ensure that when you later turn to a recipe for a digestive tea or a soothing salve, you will already know how to select fresh herbs, store them properly, measure the right amounts, and prepare them in a way that preserves their healing properties.

Most importantly, this section encourages an attitude of respect and mindfulness. Rather than rushing through the process, you will learn to observe the subtle changes in texture, aroma, and color that indicate when a tea has steeped long enough or when an oil has fully absorbed the essence of the herb. You will discover that herbalism is both an art and a science. By taking the time to understand each step, you will lay the foundation for a practice that will serve you well for years to come.

Chapter 1: Equipping Your Apothecary (Tools, Essential Equipment, Storage Solutions)

Before you begin mixing remedies, you need to gather the proper tools and materials. Think of this chapter as the foundation of your workspace. By choosing the right tools and understanding how to use them, you set yourself up for smooth preparation and consistent results. Start with a good selection of storage containers. Glass jars with tight-fitting lids are a top choice because they keep out light and moisture, helping to preserve the quality of your herbs. Brown and amber jars and bottles are especially useful for storing oils and tinctures, as they protect delicate ingredients from light degradation.

In addition to containers, invest in basic measuring tools. Teaspoons, measuring cups, and kitchen scales keep your remedies in proper proportions. Wooden spoons and bamboo whisks help you stir infusions gently without scraping the sides of containers. A mortar and pestle is invaluable for grinding dried herbs into powders. It provides more control and a connection to the herbal material that an electric grinder may lack. However, if you are working with large quantities or tough roots, a dedicated herb grinder or spice mill can be a real time saver.

Strainers and cheesecloth will prove essential for separating plant material from liquid preparations. Muslin bags can also be helpful, especially when steeping large batches of tea or infusing oils. Funnels make it easier to transfer liquids into narrow-necked bottles, and eyedroppers or pipettes allow you to measure tinctures and oils drop by drop when needed. A double boiler or a simple bowl over a pan of simmering water can gently heat oils and waxes for ointments, ensuring that delicate compounds do not burn.

For proper storage, consider a cool, dry place out of direct sunlight. Shelves lined with jars of herbs create a simple, functional apothecary that encourages you to keep track of what you have on hand. Clearly label each jar with the name of the herb, date of purchase, and any notes about its source or quality. This attention to detail will help you maintain a reliable inventory and ensure that you use your herbs before they lose their potency. Over time, you will learn which suppliers provide consistently fresh ingredients, and which regions grow the most aromatic chamomile or lavender.

As you set up your dispensary, consider creating a small reference area. Keep your notes, recipes, and any identification guides handy. This will make it easier to cross-reference information on specific herbs and document any adjustments you make to recipes. Over time, your apothecary will feel like a living library, a resource that grows richer as you gain experience.

By setting up a well-organized apothecary, you give yourself the freedom to explore remedies without frustration. This space should invite you to work methodically, so that making an ointment or mixing a tea blend becomes a soothing ritual rather than a rushed chore. With your tools assembled and your storage solutions in place, you can move on to the next steps, confident that you have built a solid foundation for all the remedies to come.

Chapter 2: Sourcing and Identifying Herbs (Foraging Basics, Ethical Harvesting, Reputable Suppliers, Growing Your Own)

The journey of herbal medicine truly begins when you know how to source and identify the plants that form the basis of your preparations. Familiarizing yourself with the natural properties of each herb will ensure that the ingredients you bring to your apothecary are both safe and effective. Start by learning the basic characteristics that distinguish one plant from another. Pay attention to leaf shape, stem texture, flower color, and aroma. Consider investing in a reliable field guide or taking a short course from a local herbalist or naturalist. The time you spend improving your identification skills will pay off in quality and confidence.

If you have access to wild areas, foraging can be a wonderful way to collect herbs directly from their natural environment. Approach this practice with care and responsibility. Check local regulations and property lines to make sure you are allowed to harvest in a particular location. Familiarize yourself with any endangered plants in your region and learn to recognize them so you can avoid disturbing their fragile populations. Harvest only what you need and never take an entire stand of a single plant. By leaving enough, you help ensure that the plants will continue to thrive and support wildlife and future foragers.

When harvesting, choose a clear, dry day and aim for late morning, when the dew has evaporated but the sun has not yet depleted the plant's vital oils. Use clean tools and handle plants gently. Shake off any insects and inspect each piece you collect for signs of disease or contamination. Store your harvest in a breathable container such as a basket or cloth bag to prevent mold from forming during transport. Once at home, process your herbs promptly by drying, freezing, or canning according to your specific needs.

Not everyone has access to wild-harvested plants, and that's okay. Reputable suppliers of dried herbs and seeds can be found through trusted herb shops, online natural marketplaces, and local farmers who grow medicinal plants. When buying herbs, ask questions about their origin, harvesting methods, and freshness. Quality suppliers will be transparent and knowledgeable, often providing lot numbers and harvest dates. Where possible, look for certifications such as organic or sustainably harvested. This helps ensure that you are getting herbs free from harmful pesticides and supports farmers who care for their land.

Another excellent option is to grow your own herbs at home. Even a small windowsill can support a few pots of culinary and medicinal plants such as mint, basil, or thyme. A garden plot or raised beds offer more possibilities, allowing you to grow a variety of herbs suited to your local climate. Growing your own not only guarantees a steady supply of fresh materials, it also deepens your understanding of how each plant changes through the seasons. You learn when to harvest leaves at their most aromatic peak or pick flowers just as they begin to open. This hands-on experience fosters a deeper connection and helps you appreciate the subtle differences in flavor and potency from one harvest to the next.

Over time, as you become more familiar with the plants you rely on, you will develop a personal network of sources. You may find a particular hillside where wild chamomile thrives in the spring, a trusted online supplier of organically grown elderberries, or a neighbor who trades fresh lavender for your dried lemon balm. By cultivating a variety of sourcing methods, you ensure that your dispensary remains well-stocked and responsive to your needs. Most importantly, remember that proper identification and ethical harvesting practices are the foundation of herbal integrity. By honoring the plants and the land from which they come, you keep alive the traditions that have guided healers for centuries.

Chapter 3: Preparation Techniques (Infusions, Decoctions, Tinctures, Oils, Vinegars, Syrups, Salves, Poultices, Oxymels, Proper Dosage)

The ability to transform raw plant materials into usable remedies is at the heart of herbal practice. By learning these techniques, you will gain the confidence to approach a wide variety of plants and unlock their healing potential. Each method extracts and preserves different qualities from the herbs, allowing you to choose the best approach for your desired outcome. To master these techniques, start by understanding their basic principles and then refine your skills through repetition and observation.

Infusions are often the easiest place to start. They involve steeping leaves and flowers in hot water to extract their aromatic oils and soluble compounds. Generally, one or two tablespoons of dried herb per cup of boiled water is a good ratio. Cover the pot while steeping to prevent valuable oils from escaping as steam. Steeping times vary, but common ranges are 5 to 15 minutes for delicate herbs and up to 30 minutes for stronger ones. Infusions are best used fresh, although they can be stored in the refrigerator for a day or two if necessary.

Decoctions apply the same principle to tougher plant materials such as roots and bark. Instead of steeping the herbs in freshly boiled water, they are simmered over low heat for 15 to 45 minutes to coax out the more resistant compounds. The result is often a stronger-tasting, more medicinal brew. When finished, strain the liquid and use it as is or add it to syrups and other preparations. Decoctions can be stored in the refrigerator for a few days, but are best consumed fresh to maintain their potency.

Tinctures rely on alcohol or glycerin to extract and preserve active compounds over time. By immersing chopped fresh or dried herbs in a solution of high-proof alcohol or a glycerin-water mixture, you create a concentrated extract that can remain stable for many months. Ratios vary, but a common guideline is to fill a jar with about one part herb to five parts alcohol. Shake the jar daily and keep it out of direct sunlight. After a few weeks, strain the liquid into dropper bottles. Tinctures are potent, so start with a small dosage and adjust as needed.

Infused oils capture the fat-soluble compounds of certain herbs. By gently warming dried plant material in a carrier oil such as olive or almond oil, you can create a base for salves, massage oils, and other topical applications. Keep the heat low to avoid scorching, and test the aroma and color as it develops. Some herbalists prefer a slow solar infusion, leaving jars of herbs and oil in a sunny window for several weeks to extract the essence without direct heat. Once strained, store your oils in dark bottles.

Vinegar-based infusions use acidic liquids such as apple cider vinegar to extract minerals and beneficial compounds, especially from nutrient-rich herbs. Steep the herbs in vinegar for a few weeks, shaking occasionally. The result can be used as a salad dressing tonic or as part of other herbal preparations. Vinegar extracts have a bright flavor and are an excellent way to incorporate herbs into everyday meals.

Syrups combine a strong infusion or decoction with a sweetener such as honey or sugar. Gently heating and stirring in the sweetener to create a thick liquid preserves the remedy and improves taste. Herbal syrups are popular for coughs, sore throats, and children's remedies because of their palatable taste. Store syrups in the refrigerator and use within a few weeks or months, depending on the recipe.

Salves are made by mixing infused oils with beeswax or vegetable wax to create a semi-solid topical preparation. The infused oil and wax are gently heated until just melted, then poured into jars or containers to solidify. Salves provide a protective and soothing barrier on the skin, making them ideal for cuts, scrapes, dry skin and sore muscles. Adjust the ratio of wax to oil to achieve the desired consistency and always test on a small patch of skin before widespread use.

Poultices use fresh or dried herbs directly on the skin. A basic poultice involves moistening ground herbs and applying them to the affected area, sometimes held in place with a cloth. Poultices deliver herbal benefits where they are needed and can be helpful in drawing out impurities or soothing irritation. Always make sure the herbs are clean and free of contaminants.

Oxymels blend honey and vinegar to create a sweet-sour base that is both pleasant and shelf stable. Steeping herbs in this mixture yields a preparation often used for respiratory or digestive support. The honey helps preserve the remedy and lessen its pungency, while the vinegar extracts valuable compounds. Dilute Oxymels in warm water or take them directly by the spoonful.

The proper dosage depends on many factors, including the potency of the herb, your individual constitution, and the nature of the ailment. Start with the recommended dosage from a trusted recipe or source and see how your body responds. Generally, infusions and decoctions are measured in cups per day, tinctures in drops or milliliters, and syrups in teaspoons. If you are unsure, start with a smaller amount and gradually increase as needed. Over time, you will develop an intuitive sense of how much is right for you.

By learning these preparation techniques, you will build a toolkit that can address a wide range of concerns. As you experiment, keep a record of what you do and the results you observe. This record will help you refine your methods by choosing the appropriate technique for each herb and situation. In the process, you will develop the adaptability that will transform you from a follower of recipes to a confident creator of your own personal remedies.

Part II: Remedies for Common Ailments.

Moving beyond basic techniques and preparations, this section of the book delves into specific remedies designed to address a wide range of common health concerns. These chapters group recipes by area of wellness, allowing you to focus on specific needs such as digestive comfort, respiratory support, or skin health. By understanding the properties of each herb and the methods best suited to unlock its healing potential, you can choose remedies that fit seamlessly into your daily life.

These preparations do not promise instant miracles, but rather steady support that encourages the body's innate ability to heal. Many of these recipes have been passed down through generations and tested over time. They respect the complexity of the body and work in harmony rather than against it. As you explore these remedies, pay attention to your own experiences. Which herbs feel most supportive to you personally? Which preparations fit easily into your routine?

It can be helpful to keep a simple journal of what you try, noting the effects, the taste, and any changes in how you feel. Over time, patterns may emerge that lead you to the remedies that resonate most strongly with your individual constitution. Remember, these are not meant to replace professional medical advice. If you have serious health concerns, always seek appropriate care. But for everyday problems, a warm cup of herbal tea or a gently applied salve can often provide comfort and relief in a natural and accessible way.

Chapter 4: Digestive Health and Metabolism (Remedies 1–40)

Our digestive system does more than just break down food. It is closely tied to our overall well-being, affecting energy levels, mood, immune function, and even the clarity of our minds. When digestion is smooth and efficient, we feel balanced and resilient. When it falters, we may experience discomfort, fatigue, or irregularities that can disrupt our daily lives. The remedies in this chapter aim to restore harmony to the digestive process, soothe irritated tissues, and promote optimal absorption of nutrients.

You will find herbs that calm inflammation, increase enzyme production, support liver function, or help maintain healthy intestinal flora. Many of these remedies are gentle enough to incorporate into your daily routine as a preventative measure. A soothing tea after a meal, a tonic first thing in the morning, or a bitters before dinner can make a noticeable difference over time. Experiment with different preparations to find those that truly nourish and support you, and consider your overall diet and lifestyle for best results. These herbs work best when combined with balanced meals, proper hydration, and mindful eating practices. Chew slowly, pay attention to hunger and satiety cues, and try to reduce overly processed foods that tax the digestive system. Together, these small changes and the traditional wisdom of these remedies can help you foster a more comfortable and resilient digestive system.

- Remedy 1: Peppermint Digestive Tonic
    - Use: Soothe mild indigestion, gas, and bloating

- Ingredients: 1 tbsp dried peppermint leaves, 1 cup hot water
- How to Prepare: Steep leaves in hot water for 10 minutes, then strain
- Tips: Sip after meals; start with a small amount if you have acid reflux

- Remedy 2: Ginger-Fennel Belly Soother
  - Use: Reduce bloating, mild nausea, and aid digestion after heavy meals
  - Ingredients: 1 tsp grated fresh ginger, 1 tsp crushed fennel seeds, 1 cup boiling water
  - How to Prepare: Steep ginger and fennel in boiling water for 10–15 minutes, then strain
  - Tips: Keep ginger root and fennel seeds on hand; adjust steep time to taste

- Remedy 3: Chamomile-Calming Tea
  - Use: Ease mild digestive discomfort and calm tension that may affect digestion
  - Ingredients: 1 tbsp dried chamomile flowers, 1 cup hot water
  - How to Prepare: Steep flowers in hot water for 5–10 minutes, then strain
  - Tips: Enjoy at the end of a long day; blend with lemon balm or mint for added calm

- Remedy 4: Bitter Orange Peel Infusion
    - Use: Stimulate digestive juices and improve digestion before meals
    - Ingredients: 1 tsp dried bitter orange peel, 1 cup just-boiled water
    - How to Prepare: Steep peel in hot water for 10 minutes, then strain and drink before meals
    - Tips: Blend with dandelion or chamomile if too bitter; experiment with steep times
- Remedy 5: Caraway Seed Digestive Aid
    - Use: Reduce gas and bloating, especially after savory meals
    - Ingredients: 1 tsp crushed caraway seeds, 1 cup hot water
    - How to Prepare: Steep seeds in hot water for 10–15 minutes, then strain
    - Tips: Add caraway seeds to cooking; store seeds in a sealed container
- Remedy 6: Cardamom Spice Tincture
    - Use: Support digestion and help relieve occasional stomach discomfort
    - Ingredients: 2 tbsp crushed cardamom pods, 1 cup high-proof alcohol

- - How to Prepare: Combine pods and alcohol in a jar, shake daily for 2 weeks, strain into dropper bottle
  - Tips: Start with a few drops before meals; store in a cool dark place
- Remedy 7: Licorice Root Stomach Ease
  - Use: Soothe irritated stomach lining and mild acid discomfort
  - Ingredients: 1 tsp dried licorice root, 1 cup hot water
  - How to Prepare: Simmer root in water for 10–15 minutes, strain
  - Tips: Use occasionally if you have high blood pressure; licorice can be sweet on its own
- Remedy 8: Turmeric-Ginger Gut Balm
  - Use: Reduce mild inflammation and support overall digestive comfort
  - Ingredients: 1 tsp grated turmeric root, 1 tsp grated ginger root, 1 cup water
  - How to Prepare: Simmer roots for 10 minutes, strain and sip warm
  - Tips: Add a pinch of black pepper for better turmeric absorption; drink after meals
- Remedy 9: Dandelion Root Bitter Elixir

- Use: Stimulate bile flow and improve fat digestion
- Ingredients: 1 tsp roasted dandelion root, 1 cup hot water
- How to Prepare: Steep root in hot water for 10–15 minutes, strain
- Tips: Enjoy 20 minutes before meals; a hint of honey can soften bitterness

- **Remedy 10: Marshmallow Root Soothing Syrup**
  - Use: Coat and soothe irritated stomach and throat tissues
  - Ingredients: 2 tbsp dried marshmallow root, 2 cups water, 1/2 cup honey
  - How to Prepare: Simmer root in water until reduced by half, strain, add honey and stir
  - Tips: Store syrup in the fridge; use a teaspoon as needed for gentle relief

- **Remedy 11: Fenugreek Bloating Relief**
  - Use: Ease gas, support healthy digestion, and soothe mild discomfort
  - Ingredients: 1 tsp fenugreek seeds, 1 cup hot water
  - How to Prepare: Steep seeds for 10–15 minutes, strain

- Tips: Slightly sweet, fenugreek pairs well with ginger; chew a few seeds after meals

- Remedy 12: Lemon Balm Stomach Tonic

    - Use: Calm nervous tension that may affect digestion and help ease mild discomfort

    - Ingredients: 1 tbsp dried lemon balm, 1 cup hot water

    - How to Prepare: Steep leaves for 5–10 minutes, strain

    - Tips: Enjoy in the evening to relax; combine with chamomile or mint

- Remedy 13: Mint-Clove Indigestion Tea

    - Use: Relieve gas, bloating, and mild cramping

    - Ingredients: 1 tbsp dried mint leaves, 2–3 whole cloves, 1 cup hot water

    - How to Prepare: Steep mint and cloves for 10 minutes, strain

    - Tips: Cloves add warmth and aroma; adjust clove amount if taste is too strong

- Remedy 14: Cinnamon Bark Digestive Powder

    - Use: Gently stimulate digestion and add warmth to meals

    - Ingredients: 1 tsp ground cinnamon bark, 1 cup hot water

- o How to Prepare: Stir cinnamon into hot water and let sit a few minutes before sipping
- o Tips: Combine with ginger or cardamom; can be sprinkled on oatmeal or added to smoothies

- Remedy 15: Gentian Root Gentle Bitter
  - o Use: Enhance digestive secretions and improve nutrient absorption
  - o Ingredients: 1 tsp dried gentian root, 1 cup hot water
  - o How to Prepare: Steep root for 10 minutes, strain
  - o Tips: Very bitter, consider mixing with orange peel or fennel for balance

- Remedy 16: Anise Seed Settling Tea
  - o Use: Ease gas, mild cramping, and promote smoother digestion
  - o Ingredients: 1 tsp crushed anise seeds, 1 cup hot water
  - o How to Prepare: Steep seeds for 10–15 minutes, strain
  - o Tips: Sweet flavor pairs well with mint; drink after meals to encourage comfort

- Remedy 17: Angelica Root Digestive Cordial

- Use: Stimulate appetite, support digestion, and ease mild discomfort
- Ingredients: 1 tbsp dried angelica root, 1 cup hot water
- How to Prepare: Simmer root for 10–15 minutes, strain
- Tips: Use before meals if appetite is low; avoid if pregnant

- Remedy 18: Holy Basil Digestive Infusion
  - Use: Support overall digestive balance and soothe mild stress-related discomfort
  - Ingredients: 1 tbsp dried holy basil leaves, 1 cup hot water
  - How to Prepare: Steep leaves 5–10 minutes, strain
  - Tips: Enjoy daily for gentle support; pairs well with lemon balm or chamomile

- Remedy 19: Rosemary Leaf Digestive Steep
  - Use: Aid circulation and mild digestive sluggishness
  - Ingredients: 1 tsp dried rosemary, 1 cup hot water
  - How to Prepare: Steep for 5–10 minutes, strain

- o Tips: Strong flavor; consider mixing with mint; enjoy before or after a meal

- Remedy 20: Coriander Seed Digestive Chai

  - o Use: Ease gas, mild cramping, and promote a comfortable belly

  - o Ingredients: 1 tsp crushed coriander seeds, 1 cup hot water

  - o How to Prepare: Steep 10–15 minutes, strain

  - o Tips: Blend with fennel or ginger; lightly sweet and aromatic

- Remedy 21: Meadowsweet Tummy Soother

  - o Use: Gently ease mild acid discomfort and calm the stomach

  - o Ingredients: 1 tbsp dried meadowsweet, 1 cup hot water

  - o How to Prepare: Steep 10 minutes, strain

  - o Tips: Contains mild salicylates; do not overuse if sensitive to aspirin

- Remedy 22: Slippery Elm Stomach Coating Brew

  - o Use: Soothe irritated tissues and support gut lining health

  - o Ingredients: 1 tsp slippery elm powder, 1 cup warm water

- o How to Prepare: Stir powder into warm water until thickened, sip slowly
- o Tips: Texture is mild and mucilaginous; add a little honey for taste

- Remedy 23: Spearmint Light Digestive Tea
  - o Use: Gently calm the stomach without strong menthol intensity
  - o Ingredients: 1 tbsp dried spearmint leaves, 1 cup hot water
  - o How to Prepare: Steep 5–10 minutes, strain
  - o Tips: Milder than peppermint; suitable for sensitive stomachs or children

- Remedy 24: Chamomile-Licorice Gut Elixir
  - o Use: Calm irritation and mild cramping while adding a soothing sweet note
  - o Ingredients: 1 tbsp chamomile, 1 tsp licorice root, 1 cup hot water
  - o How to Prepare: Steep 10 minutes, strain
  - o Tips: Mildly sweet; avoid excessive licorice if you have high blood pressure

- Remedy 25: Yarrow Digestive Support Tea
  - o Use: Stimulate digestion and assist in reducing mild bloating

- Ingredients: 1 tsp dried yarrow, 1 cup hot water
- How to Prepare: Steep 5–10 minutes, strain
- Tips: Bitter flavor; blend with mint or lemon balm to improve taste

- Remedy 26: Dill Seed Gentle Stomach Aid
  - Use: Ease gas and mild discomfort, especially after heavy meals
  - Ingredients: 1 tsp crushed dill seeds, 1 cup hot water
  - How to Prepare: Steep 10–15 minutes, strain
  - Tips: Pleasant subtle flavor; also helpful for freshening breath

- Remedy 27: Basil-Leaf Tummy Comfort Infusion
  - Use: Support mild stomach discomfort and calm occasional nausea
  - Ingredients: 1 tbsp dried basil leaves, 1 cup hot water
  - How to Prepare: Steep 5–10 minutes, strain
  - Tips: Slightly sweet and aromatic; pair with lemon balm for extra calm

- Remedy 28: Fennel-Cardamom Digestive Cordial
  - Use: Relieve bloating, mild cramping, and encourage digestive ease

- Ingredients: 1 tsp fennel seeds, 1 tsp crushed cardamom pods, 1 cup hot water
- How to Prepare: Steep 10–15 minutes, strain
- Tips: Warm, sweet-spicy flavor; soothing after rich meals

- Remedy 29: Lemon Verbena Settling Tea
    - Use: Calm mild digestive discomfort and ease tension in the belly
    - Ingredients: 1 tbsp dried lemon verbena, 1 cup hot water
    - How to Prepare: Steep 5–10 minutes, strain
    - Tips: Delicate citrus flavor; enjoy as an afternoon pick-me-up

- Remedy 30: Apple Cider Vinegar Digestive Tonic
    - Use: Support digestion by introducing gentle acidity before meals
    - Ingredients: 1 tbsp raw apple cider vinegar, 1 cup warm water
    - How to Prepare: Stir vinegar into warm water, sip before a meal
    - Tips: Add a bit of honey for taste; can help with mild sluggish digestion

- Remedy 31: Sage Leaf Light Bitter

- o Use: Stimulate digestive secretions and improve overall digestion
- o Ingredients: 1 tsp dried sage leaves, 1 cup hot water
- o How to Prepare: Steep 5–10 minutes, strain
- o Tips: Strong flavor; blend with chamomile or mint to mellow bitterness

- Remedy 32: Thyme Digestive Steep
  - o Use: Gently stimulate digestion and ease mild gas
  - o Ingredients: 1 tsp dried thyme, 1 cup hot water
  - o How to Prepare: Steep 5–10 minutes, strain
  - o Tips: Earthy flavor; combine with lemon balm for a softer taste

- Remedy 33: Bay Leaf Aromatic Tonic
  - o Use: Subtle support for digestion and mild discomfort
  - o Ingredients: 1 dried bay leaf, 1 cup hot water
  - o How to Prepare: Steep 10 minutes, strain
  - o Tips: Mildly aromatic; pair with cinnamon for extra warmth

- Remedy 34: Cinnamon-Ginger Digestive Honey

- Use: Warm the stomach and support digestion before or after meals
- Ingredients: 1 tsp cinnamon, 1 tsp grated ginger, 1 tbsp honey
- How to Prepare: Mix spices into honey; stir a spoonful into warm water
- Tips: Store honey blend in a sealed jar; soothing on cool days

- **Remedy 35: Black Pepper Digestive Spark**
  - Use: Stimulate digestive fire and improve nutrient absorption
  - Ingredients: 1/4 tsp freshly ground black pepper, 1 cup hot water
  - How to Prepare: Steep pepper for a few minutes, then strain or sip carefully
  - Tips: Strong and spicy; mix with ginger or fennel to balance heat

- **Remedy 36: Orange Peel and Clove Bitters**
  - Use: Gently prime digestion and reduce mild bloating
  - Ingredients: 1 tsp dried orange peel, 1–2 cloves, 1 cup hot water
  - How to Prepare: Steep 10 minutes, strain

- Tips: Adjust clove amount to taste; can be enjoyed before a meal

- Remedy 37: Oat Straw Gentle Stomach Infusion

    - Use: Provide soothing, mild support for overall digestion
    - Ingredients: 1 tbsp oat straw, 1 cup hot water
    - How to Prepare: Steep 10–15 minutes, strain
    - Tips: Mild taste; great combined with chamomile for a gentle blend

- Remedy 38: Chamomile-Apple Digestive Steep

    - Use: Ease mild discomfort and add a comforting flavor
    - Ingredients: 1 tbsp chamomile, a few dried apple pieces, 1 cup hot water
    - How to Prepare: Steep 10 minutes, strain
    - Tips: Lightly sweet and fragrant; pleasant evening beverage

- Remedy 39: Ginger-Mint Infused Honey

    - Use: Calm the stomach and reduce gas when stirred into warm water or tea
    - Ingredients: 1 tsp grated ginger, 1 tsp dried mint, 2 tbsp honey

- How to Prepare: Mix ginger and mint into honey; let sit a few days to infuse
- Tips: Add a spoonful to hot water as needed; store in a sealed jar

- Remedy 40: Turmeric-Lemon Digestive Water
  - Use: Encourage gentle detox and support a healthy gut environment
  - Ingredients: 1/2 tsp ground turmeric, juice of 1/2 lemon, 1 cup warm water
  - How to Prepare: Stir turmeric and lemon juice into warm water, sip slowly
  - Tips: Add a pinch of black pepper for absorption; best enjoyed in the morning

Chapter 5: Respiratory and Immune Support (Remedies 41–80)

Our respiratory and immune systems work tirelessly to keep us healthy and protected. They filter the air we breathe, defend against pathogens, and support the delicate balance that allows us to thrive. But factors such as seasonal changes, pollution, and chronic stress can strain these defenses, leading to congestion, coughing, or decreased resistance. The remedies in this chapter aim to relieve mild congestion, open the airways, and promote a robust immune response.

You will find preparations designed to soothe irritated throats, clear stuffy sinuses, and strengthen the body's natural defenses. From herbal steams that help loosen mucus to infusions that provide essential nutrients, each remedy offers a gentle step toward breathing more freely and feeling more secure against common challenges. Many of these preparations are both restorative and preventative, nourishing your body so it is better equipped to stand strong when faced with seasonal changes or environmental irritants.

As you explore these remedies, consider adopting habits that support overall wellness. Keep your living space clean and well ventilated, stay active to maintain good circulation, and choose nutrient-rich foods to strengthen your immune system from within. Combined with the thoughtful use of herbs, these simple practices will help you move toward greater vitality and protection with every breath you take.

- Remedy 41: Elderberry Immune Syrup
  - Use: Support the immune system and respiratory health during seasonal changes

- Ingredients: 1 cup dried elderberries, 4 cups water, 1 cup honey
- How to Prepare: Simmer berries in water until reduced by half, strain, add honey
- Tips: Refrigerate syrup; take by the spoonful as needed

- Remedy 42: Thyme Steam Inhalation
  - Use: Clear congestion and support healthy breathing
  - Ingredients: 1 tbsp dried thyme, bowl of hot water
  - How to Prepare: Add thyme to hot water, lean over bowl with a towel over head
  - Tips: Inhale steam for several minutes; helps soothe nasal passages

- Remedy 43: Mullein Leaf Lung Tea
  - Use: Support healthy lungs and soothe mild irritation
  - Ingredients: 1 tbsp dried mullein leaves, 1 cup hot water
  - How to Prepare: Steep 10–15 minutes, strain through a fine filter
  - Tips: Mullein can be fuzzy; strain well. Enjoy warm for gentle relief

- Remedy 44: Eucalyptus Chest Rub
    - Use: Open airways and relieve mild congestion
    - Ingredients: 1 tbsp eucalyptus-infused oil, 1 tsp beeswax
    - How to Prepare: Gently melt oil and beeswax, pour into a small tin
    - Tips: Rub on chest; keep away from eyes and face directly
- Remedy 45: Peppermint-Eucalyptus Steam Bowl
    - Use: Ease stuffy nose and promote clearer breathing
    - Ingredients: 1 tsp dried peppermint, a few drops eucalyptus oil, bowl hot water
    - How to Prepare: Add peppermint and oil to bowl, inhale steam
    - Tips: Brief sessions are best; peppermint adds a cooling sensation
- Remedy 46: Sage Gargle for Throat
    - Use: Soothe a scratchy throat and mild irritation
    - Ingredients: 1 tsp dried sage, 1 cup hot water, pinch of salt
    - How to Prepare: Steep sage in hot water, add salt, cool slightly, gargle and spit out

- - Tips: Use a few times a day as needed; do not swallow

- Remedy 47: Licorice Root Cough Ease

  - Use: Calm occasional cough and soothe throat
  - Ingredients: 1 tsp licorice root, 1 cup hot water
  - How to Prepare: Simmer root for 10–15 minutes, strain and sip
  - Tips: Do not overuse if you have high blood pressure; naturally sweet

- Remedy 48: Pine Needle Immune Tea

  - Use: Support respiratory function and gentle immune support
  - Ingredients: 1 tbsp chopped pine needles, 1 cup hot water
  - How to Prepare: Steep 10 minutes, strain
  - Tips: Ensure correct pine species; pleasant evergreen aroma

- Remedy 49: Ginger-Garlic Cold Infusion

  - Use: Warm the body, support immune response, ease mild congestion
  - Ingredients: 1 tsp grated ginger, 1 clove crushed garlic, 1 cup hot water

- - How to Prepare: Steep 10–15 minutes, strain and sip
  - Tips: Strong flavor; add honey and lemon if desired
- Remedy 50: Lemon-Honey Throat Soothe
  - Use: Coat the throat and ease mild irritation
  - Ingredients: 1 tbsp honey, juice of 1/2 lemon, 1 cup warm water
  - How to Prepare: Stir honey and lemon into warm water, sip slowly
  - Tips: Simple and effective; enjoy as needed
- Remedy 51: Marshmallow Root Throat Coating
  - Use: Soothe dry irritated throat and support easier breathing
  - Ingredients: 1 tsp marshmallow root, 1 cup warm water
  - How to Prepare: Stir root into water until slightly thick, sip slowly
  - Tips: Mild taste; add a little honey if desired
- Remedy 52: Oregano Steam Inhalation
  - Use: Support clear breathing and ease mild congestion

- Ingredients: 1 tsp dried oregano, bowl hot water
- How to Prepare: Add oregano to hot water, inhale steam under a towel
- Tips: Strong aroma; brief inhalations help clear sinuses

- **Remedy 53: Elderflower Immune Infusion**
  - Use: Support immune health and soothe mild respiratory discomfort
  - Ingredients: 1 tbsp dried elderflowers, 1 cup hot water
  - How to Prepare: Steep 10 minutes, strain
  - Tips: Delicate floral taste; combine with mint or lemon balm

- **Remedy 54: Nettle Immune Tonic**
  - Use: Nourish the body and support overall vitality during seasonal shifts
  - Ingredients: 1 tbsp dried nettle leaves, 1 cup hot water
  - How to Prepare: Steep 10–15 minutes, strain
  - Tips: Rich in nutrients; enjoy regularly for gentle support

- **Remedy 55: Rosemary Vapor Rub**

- o Use: Clear the head and encourage easier breathing
- o Ingredients: 1 tbsp rosemary-infused oil, 1 tsp beeswax
- o How to Prepare: Melt together, pour into tin, cool
- o Tips: Apply to chest or under nose sparingly

- Remedy 56: Yarrow Fever Support Tea
  - o Use: Support the body during mild fevers and encourage sweating
  - o Ingredients: 1 tsp dried yarrow, 1 cup hot water
  - o How to Prepare: Steep 10 minutes, strain
  - o Tips: Slightly bitter; blend with mint or elderflower

- Remedy 57: Chamomile Congestion Relief
  - o Use: Gently soothe nasal passages and ease mild discomfort
  - o Ingredients: 1 tbsp chamomile, 1 cup hot water
  - o How to Prepare: Steep 5–10 minutes, strain
  - o Tips: Inhale aroma as you sip; calming and soothing

- Remedy 58: Plantain Leaf Respiratory Tea

- Use: Ease mild irritation in the airways and support clear breathing
- Ingredients: 1 tbsp dried plantain leaves, 1 cup hot water
- How to Prepare: Steep 10 minutes, strain
- Tips: Mild taste; combine with peppermint or thyme

- Remedy 59: Cinnamon-Clove Warming Tonic
  - Use: Support circulation and ease mild congestion
  - Ingredients: 1/2 tsp cinnamon, 1–2 cloves, 1 cup hot water
  - How to Prepare: Steep 10 minutes, strain
  - Tips: Add honey for sweetness; warm and aromatic

- Remedy 60: Wild Cherry Bark Cough Syrup
  - Use: Ease occasional cough and soothe throat
  - Ingredients: 2 tbsp wild cherry bark, 2 cups water, 1/2 cup honey
  - How to Prepare: Simmer bark in water until reduced by half, strain, add honey
  - Tips: Store in fridge; take by the spoonful as needed

- Remedy 61: Onion-Honey Immune Syrup

    - Use: Support the body during seasonal discomfort and mild coughs

    - Ingredients: 1 small sliced onion, enough honey to cover

    - How to Prepare: Layer onion and honey in a jar, let sit overnight, strain syrup

    - Tips: Mild onion flavor; take by spoonful as needed

- Remedy 62: Echinacea Root Immune Brew

    - Use: Encourage immune response and support overall wellness

    - Ingredients: 1 tsp echinacea root, 1 cup hot water

    - How to Prepare: Simmer root 10–15 minutes, strain

    - Tips: Slightly tingly flavor; enjoy regularly during challenges

- Remedy 63: Hyssop Lung Support Infusion

    - Use: Ease mild congestion and support lung health

    - Ingredients: 1 tsp dried hyssop, 1 cup hot water

    - How to Prepare: Steep 10 minutes, strain

- o Tips: Slightly minty; combine with thyme or mullein

- Remedy 64: Lavender-Calming Vapor Bowl

    - o Use: Relax tense airways and gently clear nasal passages
    - o Ingredients: 1 tsp dried lavender, bowl hot water
    - o How to Prepare: Add lavender, inhale steam under a towel
    - o Tips: Soothing aroma; short sessions recommended

- Remedy 65: Ginger-Cayenne Warming Drink

    - o Use: Stimulate circulation, warm the body, and clear mild congestion
    - o Ingredients: 1/2 tsp grated ginger, pinch cayenne, 1 cup hot water
    - o How to Prepare: Steep ginger 10 minutes, add cayenne, strain
    - o Tips: Strong heat; add honey and lemon if desired

- Remedy 66: Fennel Seed Lung Soother

    - o Use: Gentle support for easy breathing and calm airways

- Ingredients: 1 tsp crushed fennel seeds, 1 cup hot water
- How to Prepare: Steep 10–15 minutes, strain
- Tips: Mildly sweet; combine with licorice for synergy

- Remedy 67: Elecampane Root Chest Tonic
    - Use: Support lungs and ease occasional cough
    - Ingredients: 1 tsp elecampane root, 1 cup water
    - How to Prepare: Simmer root 15 minutes, strain
    - Tips: Slight bitterness; add honey to improve taste

- Remedy 68: Lemon Balm Immune Infusion
    - Use: Calm nerves, support immunity, and ease mild tension
    - Ingredients: 1 tbsp lemon balm, 1 cup hot water
    - How to Prepare: Steep 5–10 minutes, strain
    - Tips: Pleasant citrus flavor; blend with chamomile

- Remedy 69: Tulsi (Holy Basil) Immune Steep
    - Use: Support body's resilience and balanced breathing
    - Ingredients: 1 tbsp tulsi leaves, 1 cup hot water

- - How to Prepare: Steep 5–10 minutes, strain
  - Tips: Earthy sweet flavor; enjoy daily for gradual support
- Remedy 70: Red Clover Lung Support Tea
  - Use: Gently clear airways and support overall respiratory health
  - Ingredients: 1 tbsp dried red clover blossoms, 1 cup hot water
  - How to Prepare: Steep 10 minutes, strain
  - Tips: Mild sweet taste; blend with peppermint
- Remedy 71: Horehound Cough Drops
  - Use: Ease cough and soothe throat irritation
  - Ingredients: 1 cup horehound infusion, 1 cup sugar or honey
  - How to Prepare: Simmer infusion with sweetener until thick, drop onto parchment
  - Tips: Hard candy form; store in a tin for easy use
- Remedy 72: Juniper Berry Steam
  - Use: Refresh sinuses and support clear breathing
  - Ingredients: 1 tsp crushed juniper berries, bowl hot water

- How to Prepare: Add berries to hot water, inhale steam
- Tips: Sharp aroma; short sessions recommended

- Remedy 73: Chamomile-Elderflower Chest Tea
  - Use: Gentle support for mild congestion and relaxation
  - Ingredients: 1 tsp chamomile, 1 tsp elderflower, 1 cup hot water
  - How to Prepare: Steep 10 minutes, strain
  - Tips: Floral blend; calming and soothing to sip

- Remedy 74: Peppermint-Thyme Immune Cordial
  - Use: Support breathing and mild congestion relief
  - Ingredients: 1 tsp peppermint, 1 tsp thyme, 1 cup hot water
  - How to Prepare: Steep 10 minutes, strain
  - Tips: Bright and herbal; add a bit of honey if desired

- Remedy 75: Cinnamon-Garlic Warming Broth
  - Use: Warm the body, support immunity, and ease mild congestion

- Ingredients: 1 garlic clove crushed, 1/2 tsp cinnamon, 1 cup water
- How to Prepare: Simmer 10 minutes, strain
- Tips: Unique flavor; add honey and lemon to soften taste

- Remedy 76: Astragalus Immune Decoction
  - Use: Build long-term immunity and resilience
  - Ingredients: 1 tbsp astragalus root, 2 cups water
  - How to Prepare: Simmer 20–30 minutes, strain
  - Tips: Mild taste; drink regularly in cooler seasons

- Remedy 77: Licorice-Fenugreek Throat Syrup
  - Use: Ease throat irritation and mild cough
  - Ingredients: 1 tbsp licorice root, 1 tbsp fenugreek seeds, 2 cups water, 1/2 cup honey
  - How to Prepare: Simmer herbs in water until reduced, strain, add honey
  - Tips: Store in fridge; sweet and soothing

- Remedy 78: Ginger-Thyme Honey Infusion
  - Use: Support immune function and clear mild congestion
  - Ingredients: 1 tsp grated ginger, 1 tsp thyme, 2 tbsp honey

- - How to Prepare: Mix ginger and thyme into honey; let sit, add to hot water
  - Tips: Versatile topping for tea; warming and aromatic

- Remedy 79: Clove-Lemon Immune Tonic
  - Use: Support overall wellness and gentle respiratory relief
  - Ingredients: 1–2 cloves, juice of 1/2 lemon, 1 cup hot water
  - How to Prepare: Steep cloves 10 minutes, add lemon juice, strain
  - Tips: Sharp flavor; sweeten with honey if needed

- Remedy 80: Mullein-Licorice Lung Elixir
  - Use: Soothe occasional cough and support clear breathing
  - Ingredients: 1 tbsp mullein, 1 tsp licorice root, 1 cup water
  - How to Prepare: Simmer herbs 10–15 minutes, strain
  - Tips: Strain carefully for mullein hairs; sweet note from licorice.

CHAPTER 6: SKIN AND HAIR CARE (REMEDIES 81–110)

Our skin and hair are external reflections of our internal health, creating a protective barrier and playing an important role in our appearance and self-confidence. Harsh weather, stress, poor nutrition, or exposure to irritants can challenge these protective layers, leaving them dry, brittle, or prone to irritation. The remedies in this chapter focus on restoring balance, moisturizing, soothing inflammation, and promoting a natural glow.

You will discover gentle ointments, nourishing oils, herbal rinses, and soothing compresses. These products help calm redness and dryness, add shine and strength to hair, and promote a sense of care and self-care. They rely on the natural properties of plants to maintain the integrity of our outermost layers without resorting to harsh chemicals or synthetic fragrances.

For best results, support these remedies with a balanced lifestyle. Eat a diet rich in essential fats, vitamins, and minerals. Stay hydrated, practice stress management and avoid overexposure to harsh elements. Together, these steps will help keep your skin resilient, your hair vibrant, and you confident in your own natural radiance.

- Remedy 81: Calendula Healing Salve
    - Use: Soothe minor cuts, scrapes, and dry skin
    - Ingredients: 1/4 cup calendula-infused oil, 1 tbsp beeswax

- How to Prepare: Melt oil and beeswax, pour into tin, cool
- Tips: Gentle and nourishing; test on a small area first

- Remedy 82: Aloe Vera Cooling Gel
    - Use: Calm irritated skin, minor burns, and redness
    - Ingredients: Fresh aloe vera leaf gel
    - How to Prepare: Scoop gel from leaf, apply directly
    - Tips: Store leaf in fridge for extra cooling effect

- Remedy 83: Rosewater Skin Toner
    - Use: Refresh and tone skin, reduce mild redness
    - Ingredients: Rose petals, distilled water
    - How to Prepare: Simmer petals in water, strain, cool in bottle
    - Tips: Store in fridge; use as a gentle facial mist

- Remedy 84: Lavender Moisturizing Oil
    - Use: Soften and soothe dry irritated skin
    - Ingredients: Lavender-infused oil
    - How to Prepare: Infuse dried lavender in oil, strain

- - Tips: Massage into damp skin after a bath; relaxing aroma
- Remedy 85: Chamomile Facial Steam
  - Use: Open pores, calm sensitive skin, relax facial muscles
  - Ingredients: 1 tbsp chamomile, bowl hot water
  - How to Prepare: Add chamomile to water, lean over bowl
  - Tips: Inhale gently; follow with a cool rinse
- Remedy 86: Oatmeal Soothing Bath Soak
  - Use: Relieve dry itchy skin and restore moisture
  - Ingredients: 1 cup oatmeal in a muslin bag
  - How to Prepare: Hang bag under warm bath faucet, soak
  - Tips: Gentle for all skin types; pat dry after bath
- Remedy 87: Plantain Leaf Healing Poultice
  - Use: Draw out minor irritants, soothe insect bites
  - Ingredients: Fresh plantain leaves
  - How to Prepare: Crush leaves into a paste, apply directly
  - Tips: Cover with a clean cloth; replace as needed

- Remedy 88: Comfrey Leaf Skin Compress

    - Use: Support skin healing and ease minor inflammation

    - Ingredients: Comfrey leaves, hot water

    - How to Prepare: Steep leaves, dip cloth, apply warm compress

    - Tips: Avoid use on deep wounds; short-term application only

- Remedy 89: Witch Hazel Astringent Tonic

    - Use: Tone skin, reduce excess oil, soothe mild irritation

    - Ingredients: Witch hazel extract

    - How to Prepare: Apply with cotton pad to clean skin

    - Tips: Gentle daily toner; follow with moisturizer

- Remedy 90: Rosemary Hair Rinse

    - Use: Stimulate scalp circulation, add shine

    - Ingredients: 1 tbsp dried rosemary, 2 cups hot water

    - How to Prepare: Steep, cool, pour over hair after washing

- Tips: Leave in briefly before rinsing with clean water

- Remedy 91: Hibiscus Hair Shine Infusion
  - Use: Add luster and gentle redness to hair
  - Ingredients: 1 tbsp dried hibiscus petals, 2 cups hot water
  - How to Prepare: Steep, cool, pour over hair
  - Tips: Slight tint effect; test on a small strand first

- Remedy 92: Horsetail Strengthening Hair Tea
  - Use: Support stronger hair and healthier growth
  - Ingredients: 1 tbsp dried horsetail, 2 cups hot water
  - How to Prepare: Steep, cool, rinse hair
  - Tips: Rich in silica; consistent use may show gradual results

- Remedy 93: Chamomile Brightening Hair Steep
  - Use: Naturally lighten and brighten fair hair
  - Ingredients: 1 tbsp chamomile, 2 cups hot water
  - How to Prepare: Steep, cool, rinse hair
  - Tips: Sunlight enhances effect; repeated use for subtle highlights

- Remedy 94: Nettle Hair Growth Tonic
    - Use: Support healthy scalp and encourage hair growth
    - Ingredients: 1 tbsp nettle, 2 cups hot water
    - How to Prepare: Steep, cool, rinse hair
    - Tips: Mild earthy scent; follow with light conditioner if needed
- Remedy 95: Yarrow Skin Wash
    - Use: Gently cleanse and soothe irritated skin
    - Ingredients: 1 tbsp dried yarrow, 1 cup hot water
    - How to Prepare: Steep, cool, apply with cloth
    - Tips: Mild astringent; pat skin dry afterwards
- Remedy 96: Marigold Face Mask
    - Use: Calm inflamed skin, reduce redness
    - Ingredients: 1 tbsp calendula petals, enough warm water or yogurt to form paste
    - How to Prepare: Mix petals with liquid, apply as mask, rinse after 10–15 minutes
    - Tips: Gentle on most skin types; test small area first
- Remedy 97: Rose Petal Facial Elixir

- Use: Refresh and nourish sensitive skin
- Ingredients: Fresh rose petals, light oil (almond or jojoba)
- How to Prepare: Infuse petals in oil for several weeks, strain, apply lightly
- Tips: Store in dark bottle; a few drops go a long way

- **Remedy 98: Lavender-Chamomile Bath Oil**
  - Use: Relax muscles, soften skin, and calm the mind
  - Ingredients: Lavender and chamomile-infused oil
  - How to Prepare: Add a few tablespoons to warm bath
  - Tips: Stir water to disperse oil; breathe deeply to unwind

- **Remedy 99: Peppermint Scalp Refresh Rinse**
  - Use: Cool scalp, reduce mild irritation, freshen hair
  - Ingredients: 1 tsp dried peppermint, 1 cup hot water
  - How to Prepare: Steep, cool, pour over scalp
  - Tips: Tingling sensation normal; rinse lightly if too strong

- Remedy 100: Thyme Antimicrobial Wash

    - Use: Gently cleanse minor skin irritations and support healthy skin flora

    - Ingredients: 1 tsp dried thyme, 1 cup hot water

    - How to Prepare: Steep 10 minutes, strain, cool, apply with cloth

    - Tips: Mild antiseptic properties; do not use on open wounds without caution

- Remedy 101: Honey-Lemon Face Cleanser

    - Use: Gently cleanse and brighten the complexion

    - Ingredients: 1 tsp honey, 1 tsp fresh lemon juice

    - How to Prepare: Mix honey and lemon, apply to damp skin, massage gently, rinse with warm water

    - Tips: Use once or twice a week; store honey at room temperature, use fresh lemon for best results

- Remedy 102: Sage Facial Steam

    - Use: Open pores, cleanse skin, and reduce excess oil

    - Ingredients: 1 tsp dried sage, bowl of hot water

- - How to Prepare: Add sage to hot water, lean over bowl with a towel covering your head, inhale steam for several minutes
  - Tips: Follow with a cool rinse; sage has astringent properties that help tighten pores
- Remedy 103: Mint-Cucumber Cooling Wash
  - Use: Refresh tired skin and soothe mild irritation
  - Ingredients: 1 tbsp chopped fresh mint, a few cucumber slices, 1 cup cool water
  - How to Prepare: Steep mint and cucumber in cool water for 10–15 minutes, strain, splash on face
  - Tips: Ideal on hot days; store leftover wash in the fridge for extra cooling
- Remedy 104: Calendula-Rose Facial Mist
  - Use: Tone and hydrate skin, calm mild redness
  - Ingredients: 1 tbsp calendula, 1 tbsp rose petals, 1 cup water
  - How to Prepare: Simmer petals in water, strain, cool, pour into spray bottle
  - Tips: Lightly mist face after cleansing; keep refrigerated for freshness
- Remedy 105: Chamomile-Elderflower Skin Lotion

- Use: Moisturize and soothe sensitive or dry skin
- Ingredients: 1 tbsp chamomile, 1 tbsp elderflower, 1 cup water, a few tbsp light oil, small amount beeswax
- How to Prepare: Make a strong infusion with herbs, strain, gently blend with melted beeswax and oil to form a lotion
- Tips: Adjust thickness by adding more oil or beeswax; test on a small area first

- Remedy 106: Plantain-Honey Wound Poultice
  - Use: Draw out impurities, soothe minor wounds
  - Ingredients: A few fresh plantain leaves, 1 tsp honey
  - How to Prepare: Crush plantain leaves, mix with honey, apply to clean wound, cover with gauze
  - Tips: Change poultice as needed; plantain is known for its drawing properties

- Remedy 107: Lavender-Rose Bath Salt
  - Use: Relax muscles, soften skin, and calm the mind
  - Ingredients: 1/2 cup Epsom salts, 1 tbsp dried lavender, 1 tbsp dried rose petals

- How to Prepare: Mix salts and petals, store in jar, add a handful to warm bath
- Tips: Inhale deeply while soaking; store jar tightly sealed to preserve aroma

- Remedy 108: Fenugreek Hair Conditioning Mask
  - Use: Strengthen hair and add softness
  - Ingredients: 2 tbsp fenugreek seeds, enough warm water to soak
  - How to Prepare: Soak seeds overnight, blend into paste, apply to damp hair for 20–30 minutes, rinse
  - Tips: Subtle nutty scent; use weekly for smoother hair

- Remedy 109: Basil Leaf Skin Toner
  - Use: Refresh, tone, and reduce mild blemishes
  - Ingredients: 1 tbsp dried basil, 1 cup hot water
  - How to Prepare: Steep basil 10 minutes, strain, cool, apply with cotton pad
  - Tips: Store in fridge for a few days; basil's mild antimicrobial properties can help with occasional breakouts

- Remedy 110: Rosemary-Clary Sage Hair Infusion
  - Use: Improve scalp health, add shine, and support balanced oil production

- Ingredients: 1 tsp dried rosemary, 1 tsp dried clary sage, 2 cups hot water

- How to Prepare: Steep herbs 15 minutes, strain, cool, pour over clean hair as a final rinse

- Tips: Herbal aroma lingers lightly; adjust herb amounts for your hair type

Chapter 7: Stress, Mood, and Sleep Aids (Remedies 111–140)

The pace of modern life can leave us feeling overwhelmed, anxious, or out of sync with our natural rhythms. Stress can affect not only our mood and sleep, but also our overall health and resilience. The remedies in this chapter are designed to gently bring the mind and body back into balance, promote restful sleep, relieve nervous tension, and lift the spirits during challenging times.

These preparations include calming teas, soothing infusions, aromatic pouches, and restorative tonics. These remedies work in harmony with the body's innate ability to find rest, support the nervous system, and help smooth the rough edges of daily life. They encourage you to create rituals that focus on quiet moments, slow sips, and mindful relaxation.

For lasting benefits, combine these approaches with other supportive measures. Establish a regular bedtime routine, practice deep breathing or gentle exercise, and make time for interests that rejuvenate your mind. The simple act of enjoying a warm herbal tea before bed or inhaling the subtle scent of calming herbs can help restore balance and guide you to a more peaceful state of being.

- Remedy 111: Lavender Relaxation Tea

    - Use: Calm the mind, ease mild stress, and prepare for rest

    - Ingredients: 1 tsp dried lavender, 1 cup hot water

- - How to Prepare: Steep 5–10 minutes, strain
  - Tips: Sip in the evening; combine with chamomile for extra relaxation

- Remedy 112: Lemon Balm Calm Infusion
  - Use: Reduce nervous tension and support a tranquil mood
  - Ingredients: 1 tbsp dried lemon balm, 1 cup hot water
  - How to Prepare: Steep 5–10 minutes, strain
  - Tips: Mild lemony taste; enjoy throughout the day

- Remedy 113: Passionflower Sleep Tincture
  - Use: Encourage restful sleep and ease overactive thoughts
  - Ingredients: 2 tbsp dried passionflower, 1 cup high-proof alcohol
  - How to Prepare: Infuse for 2–4 weeks, shaking daily, strain into dropper bottle
  - Tips: Start with a few drops before bed; store in a dark place

- Remedy 114: Chamomile Bedtime Tea
  - Use: Unwind at night, calm mild anxiety, and prepare for sleep

- o Ingredients: 1 tbsp dried chamomile, 1 cup hot water

- o How to Prepare: Steep 5–10 minutes, strain

- o Tips: Classic nighttime beverage; add a bit of honey if desired

- Remedy 115: Valerian Root Sleep Elixir

  - o Use: Support deeper sleep and help with occasional restlessness

  - o Ingredients: 1 tsp dried valerian root, 1 cup hot water

  - o How to Prepare: Simmer root 10–15 minutes, strain

  - o Tips: Strong aroma; start with small amounts to gauge response

- Remedy 116: Holy Basil Stress Relief Infusion

  - o Use: Help the body adapt to mild stress and enhance a sense of calm

  - o Ingredients: 1 tbsp dried holy basil, 1 cup hot water

  - o How to Prepare: Steep 5–10 minutes, strain

  - o Tips: Enjoy daily for gradual results; earthy sweet flavor

- Remedy 117: Skullcap Calming Brew

- Use: Ease nervous tension and help the mind unwind
  - Ingredients: 1 tsp dried skullcap, 1 cup hot water
  - How to Prepare: Steep 5–10 minutes, strain
  - Tips: Combine with lemon balm or chamomile for a milder taste

- Remedy 118: Rose Petal Mood Lifter
  - Use: Gently uplift mood and encourage emotional balance
  - Ingredients: 1 tbsp dried rose petals, 1 cup hot water
  - How to Prepare: Steep 5–10 minutes, strain
  - Tips: Delicate floral flavor; enjoy during quiet moments

- Remedy 119: Hops Sleep Support Tonic
  - Use: Encourage restful sleep and calm occasional tension
  - Ingredients: 1 tsp dried hops, 1 cup hot water
  - How to Prepare: Steep 5–10 minutes, strain
  - Tips: Bitter flavor; blend with chamomile or mint

- Remedy 120: Ashwagandha Restorative Steep

- Use: Support resilience, reduce mild stress, and maintain vitality
- Ingredients: 1 tsp ashwagandha root, 1 cup water
- How to Prepare: Simmer root 10–15 minutes, strain
- Tips: Earthy flavor; regular use builds benefits over time

- **Remedy 121: Linden Flower Soothing Tea**
  - Use: Gently calm nerves and encourage relaxation
  - Ingredients: 1 tbsp dried linden flowers, 1 cup hot water
  - How to Prepare: Steep 5–10 minutes, strain
  - Tips: Pleasant floral taste; sip slowly in the evening

- **Remedy 122: Peppermint-Lavender Sleep Sachet**
  - Use: Aromatic aid for restful sleep when placed near pillow
  - Ingredients: Dried peppermint and lavender flowers in a small cloth bag
  - How to Prepare: Mix equal parts herbs, fill sachet, place under pillow or beside bed

- - Tips: Replace herbs periodically for fresh scent; inhale deeply before sleep

- Remedy 123: Chamomile-Honey Night Syrup

  - Use: Calm the mind and throat for easier sleep
  - Ingredients: 1 tbsp chamomile, 1 cup water, 1/4 cup honey
  - How to Prepare: Simmer chamomile in water, strain, add honey, stir well
  - Tips: Store in fridge; take a spoonful before bed

- Remedy 124: Lavender-Lemon Foot Soak

  - Use: Relax tense muscles and soothe restless feelings before sleep
  - Ingredients: 1 tbsp dried lavender, 1 tbsp dried lemon balm, warm footbath water
  - How to Prepare: Steep herbs in hot water, add to foot basin, soak feet 15–20 minutes
  - Tips: Inhale aroma; foot soaks help signal relaxation to the whole body

- Remedy 125: St John's Wort Mood Infusion

  - Use: Support emotional balance and lift mild low spirits
  - Ingredients: 1 tsp dried St John's Wort, 1 cup hot water

- How to Prepare: Steep 5–10 minutes, strain
- Tips: Check for medication interactions; enjoy daily for cumulative effect

- Remedy 126: Saffron Uplifting Tea
  - Use: Gently brighten mood and support emotional well-being
  - Ingredients: A few saffron threads, 1 cup hot water
  - How to Prepare: Steep threads 5–10 minutes, strain
  - Tips: Subtle flavor; saffron is potent so only a few threads needed

- Remedy 127: Oat Straw Nervine Tonic
  - Use: Nourish the nervous system, reduce mild stress, and support relaxation
  - Ingredients: 1 tbsp oat straw, 1 cup hot water
  - How to Prepare: Steep 10–15 minutes, strain
  - Tips: Mild, grassy flavor; regular use supports long-term calm

- Remedy 128: Lemon Verbena Gentle Calm Tea
  - Use: Ease mild tension and foster a peaceful mind

- - Ingredients: 1 tbsp dried lemon verbena, 1 cup hot water
  - How to Prepare: Steep 5–10 minutes, strain
  - Tips: Fragrant lemony taste; enjoy in the afternoon to unwind
- Remedy 129: Chamomile-Rose Calming Blend
  - Use: Relax body and mind, reduce mild anxiety, and support restful sleep
  - Ingredients: 1 tsp chamomile, 1 tsp dried rose petals, 1 cup hot water
  - How to Prepare: Steep 5–10 minutes, strain
  - Tips: Beautiful aroma; a lovely evening ritual
- Remedy 130: Catnip Relaxation Infusion
  - Use: Calm mild restlessness and tension, support relaxation
  - Ingredients: 1 tsp dried catnip, 1 cup hot water
  - How to Prepare: Steep 5–10 minutes, strain
  - Tips: Mild minty taste; safe and gentle, especially before bed
- Remedy 131: Lavender-Elderflower Sleepy Honey
  - Use: Add gentle relaxation and flavor to bedtime teas

- Ingredients: 1 tsp dried lavender, 1 tsp elderflower, 2 tbsp honey
- How to Prepare: Mix herbs into honey, let infuse a few days, stir spoonful into warm water
- Tips: Store in a jar; floral sweetness enhances calm

- Remedy 132: Passionflower-Hops Night Cordial
  - Use: Combine calming herbs for deeper rest and easing mild insomnia
  - Ingredients: 1 tsp passionflower, 1 tsp hops, 1 cup hot water
  - How to Prepare: Steep 10 minutes, strain
  - Tips: Bitter flavor; add honey or mix with chamomile for taste

- Remedy 133: Skullcap-Valerian Rest Brew
  - Use: Stronger support for those struggling to unwind at night
  - Ingredients: 1/2 tsp skullcap, 1/2 tsp valerian, 1 cup hot water
  - How to Prepare: Steep 10–15 minutes, strain
  - Tips: Potent blend; start with small amounts to avoid grogginess

- Remedy 134: Rose-Lemon Balm Comfort Tea

- Use: Soothe mild sadness, calm nerves, and ease into rest
- Ingredients: 1 tsp rose petals, 1 tsp lemon balm, 1 cup hot water
- How to Prepare: Steep 5–10 minutes, strain
- Tips: Gentle uplifting blend; enjoy in a quiet spot

- Remedy 135: Holy Basil-Licorice Stress Support
  - Use: Adaptogenic support for mild stress and fatigue
  - Ingredients: 1 tsp holy basil, 1/2 tsp licorice root, 1 cup hot water
  - How to Prepare: Steep 10 minutes, strain
  - Tips: Sweet undertone; moderate use if concerned about blood pressure

- Remedy 136: Chamomile-Oat Straw Bedtime Blend
  - Use: Calm nervous tension and prepare for restful sleep
  - Ingredients: 1 tsp chamomile, 1 tsp oat straw, 1 cup hot water
  - How to Prepare: Steep 10 minutes, strain
  - Tips: Gentle and nourishing; sip slowly before bed

- Remedy 137: Lavender-Ginger Calm Tisane
    - Use: Relax muscles, warm the body, ease mild stress
    - Ingredients: 1 tsp lavender, 1 tsp grated ginger, 1 cup hot water
    - How to Prepare: Steep 10 minutes, strain
    - Tips: Floral-spicy flavor; adjust ginger to taste
- Remedy 138: Lemon Balm-Blue Vervain Relax Steep
    - Use: Release mild tension and encourage emotional balance
    - Ingredients: 1 tsp lemon balm, 1/2 tsp blue vervain, 1 cup hot water
    - How to Prepare: Steep 10 minutes, strain
    - Tips: Vervain is bitter; blend with chamomile if too strong
- Remedy 139: Linden-Calendula Mood Tea
    - Use: Gently uplift mood and soothe mild emotional heaviness
    - Ingredients: 1 tsp linden, 1 tsp calendula, 1 cup hot water
    - How to Prepare: Steep 5–10 minutes, strain
    - Tips: Light floral taste; enjoy regularly for subtle support

- Remedy 140: Ashwagandha-Holy Basil Night Elixir
    - Use: Support body and mind during stressful times and aid restful sleep
    - Ingredients: 1/2 tsp ashwagandha, 1 tsp holy basil, 1 cup water
    - How to Prepare: Simmer ashwagandha 10 minutes, add holy basil, steep 5 more minutes, strain
    - Tips: Earthy blend; regular use builds long-term resilience

Chapter 8: Women's Wellness and Family Health (Remedies 141–170)

Women's health and family well-being are deeply intertwined. Throughout life, different stages bring shifts in hormones, energy levels, and emotional patterns that affect everything from menstruation, fertility, and childbirth to menopause and overall vitality. The remedies in this chapter recognize these changes and offer gentle support through herbal traditions that have been trusted for generations.

Here you will find preparations to ease menstrual cramps, soothe digestive upsets in children, relieve teething, support healthy lactation, and maintain balance during menopause. These recipes do not promise instant cures, but rather steady, gentle encouragement to help the body navigate its unique journey more comfortably. They reflect the timeless wisdom passed down through families and communities, and emphasize the nurturing connection between caregivers and those they care for.

As you incorporate these remedies into your daily life, keep in mind the broader context of good nutrition, adequate rest, emotional support, and access to reliable medical care when needed. The herbs serve as allies, complementing your efforts to create a stable and loving environment in which everyone can thrive. By embracing these traditional methods, you honor the continuum of care that spans generations and cultivates resilience in body and spirit.

- Remedy 141: Raspberry Leaf Menstrual Tonic
    - Use: Support uterine health and ease mild menstrual discomfort

- Ingredients: 1 tbsp raspberry leaf, 1 cup hot water
- How to Prepare: Steep 10 minutes, strain
- Tips: Enjoy regularly before and during menstrual cycle

- **Remedy 142: Sage Hot Flash Relief Tea**
  - Use: Help ease mild hot flashes and support hormonal balance
  - Ingredients: 1 tsp dried sage, 1 cup hot water
  - How to Prepare: Steep 5–10 minutes, strain
  - Tips: Bitter flavor; add lemon balm or mint for taste

- **Remedy 143: Fenugreek Nursing Support Infusion**
  - Use: Support healthy milk production for nursing mothers
  - Ingredients: 1 tsp fenugreek seeds, 1 cup hot water
  - How to Prepare: Steep 10–15 minutes, strain
  - Tips: Sweet, nutty flavor; consult a professional if unsure

- **Remedy 144: Chamomile Children's Tummy Tea**
  - Use: Gently soothe a child's mild stomach upset

- Ingredients: 1/2 tsp chamomile, 1/2 cup hot water
- How to Prepare: Steep 5–10 minutes, strain, cool before serving
- Tips: Mild and safe in small amounts; always check temperature first

- Remedy 145: Elderflower Children's Immunity Syrup
  - Use: Support overall well-being and gentle immune function for children
  - Ingredients: 1 tbsp elderflowers, 1 cup water, 1/4 cup honey
  - How to Prepare: Simmer flowers in water, strain, add honey
  - Tips: Give small spoonfuls as needed; store in fridge

- Remedy 146: Red Clover Menopause Support
  - Use: Gently assist in balancing hormones during menopause
  - Ingredients: 1 tbsp red clover, 1 cup hot water
  - How to Prepare: Steep 10 minutes, strain
  - Tips: Mildly sweet; drink regularly for cumulative benefit

- Remedy 147: Nettle Iron-Rich Tea

- Use: Boost iron and minerals important for women's health
- Ingredients: 1 tbsp nettle, 1 cup hot water
- How to Prepare: Steep 10–15 minutes, strain
- Tips: Rich, green flavor; drink regularly for nourishment

- **Remedy 148: Motherwort Calming Tonic**
  - Use: Ease mild anxiety and tension associated with hormonal changes
  - Ingredients: 1 tsp motherwort, 1 cup hot water
  - How to Prepare: Steep 10 minutes, strain
  - Tips: Bitter taste; blend with lemon balm or mint

- **Remedy 149: Fennel Seed Nursing Aid**
  - Use: Support milk flow and soothe mild digestive discomfort in nursing mothers
  - Ingredients: 1 tsp fennel seeds, 1 cup hot water
  - How to Prepare: Steep 10–15 minutes, strain
  - Tips: Subtle sweet flavor; enjoy after nursing sessions

- **Remedy 150: Lemon Balm Children's Calming Infusion**
  - Use: Gently calm nervous children and settle mild restlessness

- Ingredients: 1 tsp lemon balm, 1 cup hot water
- How to Prepare: Steep 5–10 minutes, strain, cool before giving to child
- Tips: Mild taste; ensure appropriate age and dosage

- Remedy 151: Ginger Pregnancy Nausea Tea
  - Use: Ease mild nausea during early pregnancy
  - Ingredients: 1 tsp grated fresh ginger, 1 cup hot water
  - How to Prepare: Steep 10 minutes, strain
  - Tips: Sip slowly; check with a healthcare provider first

- Remedy 152: Raspberry Leaf Uterine Tonic
  - Use: Tone uterine muscles and support overall reproductive health
  - Ingredients: 1 tbsp raspberry leaf, 1 cup hot water
  - How to Prepare: Steep 10 minutes, strain
  - Tips: Regular use recommended; traditionally used late in pregnancy

- Remedy 153: Calendula Sitz Bath
  - Use: Soothe postpartum discomfort and support gentle healing

- Ingredients: 1–2 tbsp calendula petals, warm sitz bath water
    - How to Prepare: Steep petals in hot water, add to sitz bath
    - Tips: Relax for 10–20 minutes; gentle and calming
- Remedy 154: Chamomile Teething Soother
    - Use: Calm a teething infant's mild discomfort
    - Ingredients: 1/2 tsp chamomile, 1/2 cup hot water
    - How to Prepare: Steep 5–10 minutes, cool, dab on gums with clean cloth
    - Tips: Check temperature; small amounts only
- Remedy 155: Oat Straw Mineral-Rich Infusion
    - Use: Provide essential minerals for overall female health
    - Ingredients: 1 tbsp oat straw, 1 cup hot water
    - How to Prepare: Steep 10–15 minutes, strain
    - Tips: Regular use improves nutrition; mild taste
- Remedy 156: Lavender Child Sleep Spray
    - Use: Help children relax at bedtime with a soothing scent

- Ingredients: Lavender hydrosol or diluted lavender essential oil in water
    - How to Prepare: Mix solution in spray bottle, lightly mist bedding
    - Tips: Keep scent mild; always test for sensitivity
- Remedy 157: Rose Petal Fertility Steep
    - Use: Create a supportive environment for women trying to conceive
    - Ingredients: 1 tbsp dried rose petals, 1 cup hot water
    - How to Prepare: Steep 5–10 minutes, strain
    - Tips: Gentle and symbolic; combine with a balanced lifestyle
- Remedy 158: Hawthorn Berry Supportive Tea
    - Use: Strengthen overall health and gentle circulatory support for women
    - Ingredients: 1 tsp hawthorn berries, 1 cup hot water
    - How to Prepare: Simmer berries 10–15 minutes, strain
    - Tips: Mild fruity flavor; long-term use recommended
- Remedy 159: Marshmallow Root Children's Throat Syrup

- Use: Soothe irritated throat in children
- Ingredients: 1 tsp marshmallow root, 1 cup water, 1/4 cup honey
- How to Prepare: Simmer root, reduce, strain, add honey
- Tips: Mild and sweet; use by teaspoon as needed

- Remedy 160: Sage Menopause Balance Tisane
    - Use: Help regulate mild mood swings and hot flashes
    - Ingredients: 1 tsp sage, 1 cup hot water
    - How to Prepare: Steep 5–10 minutes, strain
    - Tips: Blend with lemon balm for better flavor

- Remedy 161: Chasteberry Hormone Balancer
    - Use: Support hormonal balance in women's cycles
    - Ingredients: 1 tsp chasteberry, 1 cup water
    - How to Prepare: Simmer berries 10–15 minutes, strain
    - Tips: Long-term use often recommended; consult professional if unsure

- Remedy 162: Peppermint Pregnancy Comfort Tea

- o Use: Ease mild nausea and occasional discomfort in pregnancy
- o Ingredients: 1 tsp peppermint, 1 cup hot water
- o How to Prepare: Steep 5–10 minutes, strain
- o Tips: Mild and refreshing; check with provider first

- Remedy 163: Red Raspberry Leaf Postpartum Tonic
  - o Use: Support recovery and replenish nutrients after childbirth
  - o Ingredients: 1 tbsp raspberry leaf, 1 cup hot water
  - o How to Prepare: Steep 10 minutes, strain
  - o Tips: Enjoy daily; combines well with nettle or oat straw

- Remedy 164: Lemon Balm Family Stress Tea
  - o Use: Calm mild tension for the whole family
  - o Ingredients: 1 tbsp lemon balm, 1 cup hot water
  - o How to Prepare: Steep 5–10 minutes, strain
  - o Tips: Mild, pleasant taste; suitable for older children in moderation

- Remedy 165: Fennel-Cardamom Nursing Biscuit
  - o Use: Gentle digestive support and mild lactation aid

- Ingredients: Ground fennel, ground cardamom, flour, honey, butter
- How to Prepare: Mix spices into biscuit dough, bake, enjoy as snack
- Tips: Subtle flavor; a comforting treat for nursing mothers

- **Remedy 166: Chamomile-Licorice Children's Cough Tea**
  - Use: Soothe mild cough and calm a restless child
  - Ingredients: 1/2 tsp chamomile, pinch licorice root, 1/2 cup hot water
  - How to Prepare: Steep 5–10 minutes, strain, cool
  - Tips: Mildly sweet; use sparingly with licorice

- **Remedy 167: Rosehip Vitamin C Infusion**
  - Use: Boost vitamin C intake and support overall health
  - Ingredients: 1 tsp crushed rosehips, 1 cup hot water
  - How to Prepare: Steep 10–15 minutes, strain
  - Tips: Tart flavor; add honey if desired

- **Remedy 168: Lavender-Oat Bath Soak for Children**

- Use: Calm and soothe children before bed
- Ingredients: 1 tbsp dried lavender, 1/2 cup oatmeal in a cloth bag
- How to Prepare: Hang bag under warm running bath water
- Tips: Gentle and skin-friendly; supervise child at all times

- Remedy 169: Parsley Leaf Mineral Tea
  - Use: Provide gentle mineral support for overall wellness
  - Ingredients: 1 tsp dried parsley, 1 cup hot water
  - How to Prepare: Steep 5–10 minutes, strain
  - Tips: Slightly grassy flavor; regular use for best effect

- Remedy 170: Skullcap Hormone Support Infusion
  - Use: Ease mild stress and tension associated with hormonal cycles
  - Ingredients: 1 tsp skullcap, 1 cup hot water
  - How to Prepare: Steep 5–10 minutes, strain
  - Tips: Blend with chamomile if taste too bitter

Chapter 9: Joint, Muscle, and Mobility Support (Remedies 171–200)

Healthy joints and muscles are the foundation of our mobility, allowing us to move through life with ease and independence. Over time, wear and tear, injury, poor posture, or inflammation can cause stiffness, discomfort, or limited range of motion. The remedies in this chapter are designed to relieve minor aches and pains, support flexibility, and help maintain the fluidity and strength essential for daily activities.

You will find balms, infused oils, warming compresses, and teas rich in beneficial compounds. These preparations harness the power of plants known to relieve discomfort, improve circulation, and promote tissue resilience. They work best when integrated into a comprehensive approach that includes regular exercise, gentle stretching, and a balanced diet, all of which help keep the body limber and well aligned.

Consider adopting simple habits such as warming up before exercise, taking breaks when sitting for long periods, and paying attention to ergonomics at home and at work. By combining these practices with time-honored herbal support, you create a sustainable pattern that can maintain your joint and muscle health, allowing you to stay active and engaged in the pursuits that bring joy and fulfillment.

- Remedy 171: Turmeric Anti-Inflammatory Paste

    o Use: Support joint comfort and reduce mild inflammation

    o Ingredients: 2 tbsp ground turmeric, water, 1 tbsp coconut oil, pinch black pepper

- - How to Prepare: Simmer turmeric and water into a paste, add oil and pepper
  - Tips: Add paste to warm milk or tea; store in fridge short-term
- Remedy 172: Willow Bark Joint Decoction
  - Use: Ease mild joint aches and tension
  - Ingredients: 1 tsp willow bark, 1 cup water
  - How to Prepare: Simmer 10–15 minutes, strain
  - Tips: Contains salicylates; use moderately
- Remedy 173: Comfrey Leaf Poultice
  - Use: Support minor sprains and ease muscle tension
  - Ingredients: Fresh comfrey leaves, a little warm water
  - How to Prepare: Mash leaves into paste, apply to affected area
  - Tips: Short-term external use only; do not use on open wounds
- Remedy 174: Arnica Muscle Rub
  - Use: Ease soreness, bruises, and minor aches
  - Ingredients: Arnica-infused oil, beeswax
  - How to Prepare: Melt beeswax into oil, pour into tin

- o Tips: External use only; test on small area first

- Remedy 175: Ginger-Cayenne Warming Compress

    - o Use: Improve circulation and ease stiff joints
    - o Ingredients: 1 tsp grated ginger, pinch cayenne, warm water and cloth
    - o How to Prepare: Steep ginger and cayenne in warm water, soak cloth, apply
    - o Tips: Check skin sensitivity; warmth helps relieve stiffness

- Remedy 176: St John's Wort Massage Oil

    - o Use: Relax tense muscles and soothe mild nerve discomfort
    - o Ingredients: St John's Wort-infused oil
    - o How to Prepare: Massage into sore areas gently
    - o Tips: Use in evening; store oil in dark bottle

- Remedy 177: Devil's Claw Joint Tonic

    - o Use: Support comfortable joints and mild mobility issues
    - o Ingredients: 1 tsp devil's claw root, 1 cup water
    - o How to Prepare: Simmer root 10–15 minutes, strain
    - o Tips: Bitter flavor; regular use recommended

- Remedy 178: Chamomile Muscle Soak
    - Use: Relax tired muscles and calm tension
    - Ingredients: 1/4 cup chamomile, bathwater
    - How to Prepare: Steep chamomile in hot water, add to bath
    - Tips: Inhale aroma; soak 15–20 minutes
- Remedy 179: Nettle Anti-Inflammatory Infusion
    - Use: Provide minerals and mild anti-inflammatory support
    - Ingredients: 1 tbsp nettle, 1 cup hot water
    - How to Prepare: Steep 10–15 minutes, strain
    - Tips: Regular use supports overall resilience
- Remedy 180: Ashwagandha Joint Steep
    - Use: Build long-term support for joint and muscle comfort
    - Ingredients: 1 tsp ashwagandha root, 1 cup water
    - How to Prepare: Simmer root 10–15 minutes, strain
    - Tips: Earthy taste; consistent use recommended
- Remedy 181: White Willow Bark Tea

- Use: Ease mild aches in joints and muscles
- Ingredients: 1 tsp willow bark, 1 cup water
- How to Prepare: Simmer 10–15 minutes, strain
- Tips: Similar to aspirin; moderate intake

- Remedy 182: Rosemary-Cayenne Liniment
  - Use: Stimulate circulation and warm sore muscles
  - Ingredients: Rosemary-infused oil, cayenne powder, small amount beeswax
  - How to Prepare: Warm and blend, strain into tin
  - Tips: Test on small area; wash hands after use

- Remedy 183: Horsetail Mineral Joint Tisane
  - Use: Supply silica and support connective tissue health
  - Ingredients: 1 tsp horsetail, 1 cup hot water
  - How to Prepare: Steep 10–15 minutes, strain
  - Tips: Regular use helps strengthen tissues

- Remedy 184: Peppermint Cooling Muscle Rub
  - Use: Ease tension with a cooling sensation
  - Ingredients: Peppermint-infused oil, beeswax

- How to Prepare: Melt beeswax into oil, pour into tin
- Tips: Great after exercise; avoid eyes

- Remedy 185: Meadowsweet Joint Comfort Tea
  - Use: Reduce mild discomfort in joints and muscles
  - Ingredients: 1 tsp meadowsweet, 1 cup hot water
  - How to Prepare: Steep 10–15 minutes, strain
  - Tips: Contains salicylates; mild, soothing taste

- Remedy 186: Turmeric-Ginger Mobility Tincture
  - Use: Support flexibility and reduce mild stiffness
  - Ingredients: Equal parts grated turmeric and ginger, high-proof alcohol
  - How to Prepare: Infuse 2–4 weeks, strain
  - Tips: Take a few drops daily; store in dark place

- Remedy 187: Birch Leaf Soothing Compress
  - Use: Relieve mild swelling and ease soreness
  - Ingredients: 1 tbsp dried birch leaves, hot water, cloth
  - How to Prepare: Steep leaves, soak cloth, apply warm compress

- Tips: Refresh as needed; relaxing and gentle
- Remedy 188: Valerian Muscle Relax Tea
    - Use: Relax tense muscles and ease mild spasms
    - Ingredients: 1 tsp valerian root, 1 cup hot water
    - How to Prepare: Simmer root 10–15 minutes, strain
    - Tips: Strong aroma; best used at night
- Remedy 189: Pine Needle Circulation Bath
    - Use: Stimulate circulation and refresh tired limbs
    - Ingredients: Handful of pine needles, hot bathwater
    - How to Prepare: Steep needles in hot water, add to bath
    - Tips: Invigorating aroma; soak 15–20 minutes
- Remedy 190: Lavender Joint Massage Oil
    - Use: Gently ease tension and mild soreness in joints
    - Ingredients: Lavender-infused oil
    - How to Prepare: Massage gently into affected areas
    - Tips: Relaxing scent; apply after warm compress

- Remedy 191: Boswellia Resin Joint Support
    - Use: Support comfortable movement and reduce mild inflammation
    - Ingredients: Boswellia resin powder, hot water
    - How to Prepare: Simmer a pinch of powder 10–15 minutes, strain
    - Tips: Earthy taste; consistent use recommended
- Remedy 192: Ginger-Turmeric Honey Blend
    - Use: Add mild anti-inflammatory and warming benefits to drinks
    - Ingredients: 1 tsp grated ginger, 1 tsp turmeric, 2 tbsp honey
    - How to Prepare: Mix thoroughly, let infuse, stir into warm water or tea
    - Tips: Store in sealed jar; enjoy daily
- Remedy 193: Thyme Warming Muscle Oil
    - Use: Improve circulation and relieve mild stiffness
    - Ingredients: Thyme-infused oil
    - How to Prepare: Massage into sore areas
    - Tips: Pleasant herbal scent; use after a warm shower

- Remedy 194: Yarrow Joint Bath Infusion
    - Use: Soothe achy joints and relax muscles
    - Ingredients: 1–2 tbsp yarrow, hot bathwater
    - How to Prepare: Steep yarrow in hot water, add to bath
    - Tips: Lightly floral scent; soak 15–20 minutes
- Remedy 195: Licorice Root Anti-Inflammatory Brew
    - Use: Gently ease mild inflammation and discomfort
    - Ingredients: 1 tsp licorice root, 1 cup water
    - How to Prepare: Simmer 10–15 minutes, strain
    - Tips: Sweet taste; moderate use if blood pressure concerns
- Remedy 196: Mullein Leaf Joint Tonic
    - Use: Soothe mild stiffness and promote easier movement
    - Ingredients: 1 tbsp mullein leaves, 1 cup hot water
    - How to Prepare: Steep 10–15 minutes, strain well
    - Tips: Mild flavor; combine with ginger for warmth
- Remedy 197: Chamomile-Hops Muscle Ease Tea

- Use: Relax tense muscles and calm the mind
- Ingredients: 1 tsp chamomile, 1 tsp hops, 1 cup hot water
- How to Prepare: Steep 10 minutes, strain
- Tips: Evening use recommended; aids relaxation

- Remedy 198: Clove Warming Liniment
  - Use: Increase blood flow and relieve mild soreness
  - Ingredients: Clove-infused oil, beeswax
  - How to Prepare: Melt wax into oil, cool in tin
  - Tips: Strong aroma; test small area first

- Remedy 199: Fenugreek Joint Comfort Steep
  - Use: Ease mild joint discomfort and support overall wellness
  - Ingredients: 1 tsp fenugreek seeds, 1 cup hot water
  - How to Prepare: Steep 10–15 minutes, strain
  - Tips: Nutty taste; add honey if desired

- Remedy 200: Cat's Claw Joint Support Infusion
  - Use: Encourage flexibility and ease mild swelling

- Ingredients: 1 tsp cat's claw bark, 1 cup water
- How to Prepare: Simmer 10–15 minutes, strain
- Tips: Earthy flavor; steady use may yield long-term benefits

Chapter 10: Energy and Vitality (Remedies 201–220)

Vibrant energy and sustained vitality are not just about avoiding disease. They come from feeling engaged, enthusiastic, and nourished by the world around us. The demands of life can sometimes deplete our reserves, leaving us tired or unmotivated. The remedies in this chapter offer gentle encouragement to restore stamina, sharpen focus, and cultivate consistent energy throughout the day.

You will find herbs and supplements that support metabolic function, enhance mental clarity, and build stamina. These are not quick fixes, but long-term allies that help you maintain a balanced internal environment. By gently enhancing the body's natural rhythms, these remedies can help you feel more capable and resilient in the face of daily challenges.

To support their effects, maintain a nutritious diet, regular physical activity, and adequate rest. Reduce factors that deplete energy, such as poor sleep patterns or nutrient-poor meals. Over time, these herbal supports combined with healthy choices will help you feel more dynamically alert and able to meet your responsibilities with a sense of confidence and well-being.

- Remedy 201: Ginseng Vitality Tonic

    - Use: Enhance overall energy, support stamina, and reduce mild fatigue

    - Ingredients: 1 tsp dried ginseng root, 1 cup water

- - How to Prepare: Simmer root for 10–15 minutes, strain
  - Tips: Earthy flavor; regular use can help build long-term vitality
- Remedy 202: Gotu Kola Focus Infusion
  - Use: Support mental clarity, concentration, and a balanced mood
  - Ingredients: 1 tsp gotu kola leaves, 1 cup hot water
  - How to Prepare: Steep 5–10 minutes, strain
  - Tips: Mildly herbal taste; daily use may improve focus over time
- Remedy 203: Matcha Green Energy Blend
  - Use: Gentle caffeine boost, antioxidants, and mental alertness
  - Ingredients: 1/2 tsp matcha powder, 1 cup hot water
  - How to Prepare: Whisk matcha into hot water until frothy
  - Tips: Start with small amounts if new to caffeine; smooth, grassy flavor
- Remedy 204: Maca Root Energy Elixir
  - Use: Support endurance, mild hormonal balance, and sustained energy

- Ingredients: 1 tsp maca powder, warm milk or water
- How to Prepare: Stir powder into warm liquid until dissolved
- Tips: Nutty flavor; add honey or cocoa for taste, enjoy regularly

- Remedy 205: Astragalus Rejuvenation Brew
  - Use: Promote resilience, immune support, and gentle energy uplift
  - Ingredients: 1 tsp astragalus root, 1 cup water
  - How to Prepare: Simmer 20–30 minutes, strain
  - Tips: Subtle sweetness; daily use supports overall well-being

- Remedy 206: Rhodiola Vitality Infusion
  - Use: Adaptogenic support for stress-related fatigue and improved stamina
  - Ingredients: 1 tsp rhodiola root, 1 cup water
  - How to Prepare: Simmer root 10–15 minutes, strain
  - Tips: Slightly bitter; regular use helps maintain balanced energy

- Remedy 207: Holy Basil Adaptogenic Tea

- Use: Enhance mental clarity, reduce mild stress, and improve energy levels
- Ingredients: 1 tbsp holy basil, 1 cup hot water
- How to Prepare: Steep 5–10 minutes, strain
- Tips: Earthy sweet flavor; consistent use encourages steady vitality

- **Remedy 208: Schisandra Berry Energy Cordial**
  - Use: Improve focus, endurance, and mild stress adaptation
  - Ingredients: 1 tsp schisandra berries, 1 cup water
  - How to Prepare: Simmer berries 10–15 minutes, strain
  - Tips: Tart and complex flavor; consider adding honey for sweetness

- **Remedy 209: Rosemary Mental Clarity Tea**
  - Use: Stimulate circulation to the head, improve alertness
  - Ingredients: 1 tsp dried rosemary, 1 cup hot water
  - How to Prepare: Steep 5–10 minutes, strain
  - Tips: Strong flavor; blend with lemon balm if taste too pungent

- Remedy 210: Lemon Balm Gentle Uplift Infusion
    - Use: Lightly boost mood, reduce mild tension, and support steady energy
    - Ingredients: 1 tbsp lemon balm, 1 cup hot water
    - How to Prepare: Steep 5–10 minutes, strain
    - Tips: Pleasant lemony flavor; enjoy as a mid-afternoon pick-me-up
- Remedy 211: Nettle Mineral-Rich Steep
    - Use: Provide minerals and gentle revitalization, improve steady energy
    - Ingredients: 1 tbsp nettle, 1 cup hot water
    - How to Prepare: Steep 10–15 minutes, strain
    - Tips: Green, grassy taste; regular use supports overall vitality
- Remedy 212: Licorice Root Vitality Brew
    - Use: Mild adrenal support, gentle energy lift, and balanced stamina
    - Ingredients: 1 tsp licorice root, 1 cup water
    - How to Prepare: Simmer 10–15 minutes, strain
    - Tips: Sweet flavor; moderate use if blood pressure concerns
- Remedy 213: Hibiscus Revitalizing Tea

- Use: Refresh and energize with vitamin C and antioxidants
- Ingredients: 1 tbsp dried hibiscus petals, 1 cup hot water
- How to Prepare: Steep 5–10 minutes, strain
- Tips: Tart, cranberry-like flavor; enjoy iced or warm

- Remedy 214: Bee Pollen Energy Blend
  - Use: Nutrient-rich boost, support endurance and mild fatigue relief
  - Ingredients: 1 tsp bee pollen, warm water or juice
  - How to Prepare: Stir pollen into liquid until mixed
  - Tips: Start with small amounts; store in a cool place

- Remedy 215: Rosehip Vitamin Tea
  - Use: Provide natural vitamin C, support steady energy and immunity
  - Ingredients: 1 tsp crushed rosehips, 1 cup hot water
  - How to Prepare: Steep 10–15 minutes, strain
  - Tips: Tangy flavor; add honey if desired

- Remedy 216: Ginkgo Leaf Clarity Infusion

    - Use: Support circulation to the brain, enhance focus and alertness

    - Ingredients: 1 tsp ginkgo leaves, 1 cup hot water

    - How to Prepare: Steep 5–10 minutes, strain

    - Tips: Mildly bitter; blend with mint or lemon balm for taste

- Remedy 217: Moringa Nutrient-Rich Brew

    - Use: Provide vitamins, minerals, and mild energy support

    - Ingredients: 1 tsp moringa leaf powder, 1 cup hot water

    - How to Prepare: Stir powder into hot water, steep a few minutes, strain if needed

    - Tips: Slightly spinach-like flavor; enjoy daily for gentle nourishment

- Remedy 218: Cinnamon-Cacao Energy Tonic

    - Use: Warm circulation, provide gentle mood lift and mild stimulant effect

    - Ingredients: 1 tsp cacao nibs, 1/2 tsp cinnamon, 1 cup hot water

    - How to Prepare: Steep nibs and cinnamon 10 minutes, strain

- o Tips: Rich and warming; add honey or milk for comfort

- Remedy 219: Dandelion Root Mineral Coffee

    - o Use: Coffee alternative, support liver health, provide mild energy
    - o Ingredients: 1 tsp roasted dandelion root, 1 cup hot water
    - o How to Prepare: Simmer root 10–15 minutes, strain
    - o Tips: Earthy flavor; add milk or cinnamon for taste

- Remedy 220: Cordyceps Mushroom Vitality Steep

    - o Use: Enhance endurance, support energy, and physical resilience
    - o Ingredients: 1 tsp dried cordyceps, 1 cup water
    - o How to Prepare: Simmer 15–20 minutes, strain
    - o Tips: Mild earthy flavor; regular use builds long-term benefits

Chapter 11: Seasonal Tonics and Year-Round Wellbeing (Remedies 221–235)

The world around us changes with each season, bringing shifts in temperature, humidity, and available food. Our bodies respond to these cycles by adjusting our metabolism, energy levels, and even our emotional landscape. The remedies in this chapter embrace the rhythms of nature, offering support to adapt to the unique demands of each season and ensure year-round resilience.

You will find cleansing tonics for spring, cooling teas for summer, immune boosters for fall, and warming drinks for winter. These preparations help you navigate seasonal transitions more gracefully, smoothing the adjustments your body makes as the environment changes. They encourage you to live in harmony with the natural flow of time, rather than resisting it.

Combine these remedies with seasonal habits such as enjoying fresh produce when it is ripe, dressing appropriately for the weather, and creating rituals that celebrate each season. In this way, you foster a lifestyle rooted in awareness, adaptability, and gratitude. Through this approach, you bring the wisdom of nature into your daily life, nurturing a vitality that endures through the changing seasons.

- Remedy 221: Spring Dandelion Cleansing Infusion

    o Use: Gently support seasonal detox and refresh energy in spring

    o Ingredients: 1 tbsp dandelion leaves, 1 cup hot water

- - How to Prepare: Steep 10 minutes, strain
  - Tips: Slightly bitter; combine with mint for flavor
- Remedy 222: Spring Nettle Mineral Tonic
  - Use: Replenish nutrients as seasons change, support vitality
  - Ingredients: 1 tbsp nettle, 1 cup hot water
  - How to Prepare: Steep 10–15 minutes, strain
  - Tips: Drink regularly for steady mineral intake
- Remedy 223: Summer Mint-Hibiscus Cooling Tea
  - Use: Cool the body, stay hydrated, and refresh during hot weather
  - Ingredients: 1 tsp mint, 1 tsp hibiscus, 1 cup hot water
  - How to Prepare: Steep 5–10 minutes, strain, serve iced if desired
  - Tips: Tart and minty; perfect summer refresher
- Remedy 224: Summer Rose Petal Hydration Infusion
  - Use: Lightly flavor water and encourage gentle relaxation in warm months
  - Ingredients: 1 tbsp dried rose petals, 1 cup hot water

- - How to Prepare: Steep 5–10 minutes, strain, serve warm or chilled
  - Tips: Delicate floral taste; add lemon for brightness
- Remedy 225: Autumn Elderberry Immune Cordial
  - Use: Support immunity during seasonal transitions
  - Ingredients: 1 tbsp dried elderberries, 1 cup water, honey to taste
  - How to Prepare: Simmer berries until reduced by half, strain, add honey
  - Tips: Store in fridge; spoonful daily as seasons shift
- Remedy 226: Autumn Apple-Cinnamon Warming Tea
  - Use: Comfort and warm the body as weather cools
  - Ingredients: Apple slices, 1/2 tsp cinnamon, 1 cup hot water
  - How to Prepare: Steep cinnamon and apples 10 minutes, strain
  - Tips: Sweet and warming; perfect for crisp fall days
- Remedy 227: Winter Ginger-Clove Warming Syrup

- Use: Support warmth and circulation in cold months
- Ingredients: 1 tsp grated ginger, a few cloves, 1 cup water, honey
- How to Prepare: Simmer spices, strain, add honey, store in fridge
- Tips: Stir into hot water for a comforting winter drink

- Remedy 228: Winter Thyme Immunity Steep
  - Use: Support resilience and breathing in colder season
  - Ingredients: 1 tsp dried thyme, 1 cup hot water
  - How to Prepare: Steep 10 minutes, strain
  - Tips: Herbal and savory; add honey or lemon if desired

- Remedy 229: Seasonal Lemon-Honey Tonic
  - Use: Keep a versatile tonic for all seasons to support well-being
  - Ingredients: Juice of 1/2 lemon, 1 tbsp honey, 1 cup warm water
  - How to Prepare: Stir honey and lemon into warm water
  - Tips: Enjoy year-round for gentle immune and digestive support

- Remedy 230: Seasonal Sage-Thyme Chest Brew
    - Use: Support clear breathing and mild congestion relief anytime
    - Ingredients: 1 tsp sage, 1 tsp thyme, 1 cup hot water
    - How to Prepare: Steep 10 minutes, strain
    - Tips: Herbal and slightly bitter; add mint for flavor
- Remedy 231: Seasonal Lavender Relaxation Tea
    - Use: Calm nerves and promote restful moments year-round
    - Ingredients: 1 tsp lavender, 1 cup hot water
    - How to Prepare: Steep 5–10 minutes, strain
    - Tips: Pair with chamomile anytime tension arises
- Remedy 232: Seasonal Chamomile Nourishing Infusion
    - Use: Gentle wellness support through changing seasons
    - Ingredients: 1 tbsp chamomile, 1 cup hot water
    - How to Prepare: Steep 5–10 minutes, strain
    - Tips: Mild and comforting; combine with other seasonal herbs

- Remedy 233: Seasonal Oat Straw Balancing Brew
    - Use: Provide minerals and steady support throughout the year
    - Ingredients: 1 tbsp oat straw, 1 cup hot water
    - How to Prepare: Steep 10–15 minutes, strain
    - Tips: Neutral flavor; enjoy daily for subtle nourishment
- Remedy 234: Seasonal Peppermint Comfort Steep
    - Use: Refresh the senses and ease mild seasonal discomfort
    - Ingredients: 1 tbsp peppermint, 1 cup hot water
    - How to Prepare: Steep 5–10 minutes, strain
    - Tips: Cooling in summer, soothing in winter; versatile year-round
- Remedy 235: Seasonal Rosemary Invigorating Infusion
    - Use: Stimulate circulation and alertness any time of year
    - Ingredients: 1 tsp dried rosemary, 1 cup hot water
    - How to Prepare: Steep 5–10 minutes, strain
    - Tips: Strong flavor; blend with lemon balm or mint

Chapter 12: Kitchen Apothecary (Remedies 236–245)

Your kitchen can be much more than a place to prepare meals. With the right knowledge, it can be transformed into a home apothecary, stocked with familiar ingredients that double as healing allies. The remedies in this chapter demonstrate how everyday foods, herbs, and spices can serve both culinary pleasures and gentle therapeutic purposes.

You will discover syrups, vinegars, honeys, and spice blends that offer subtle benefits when incorporated into your meals or taken by the spoonful. These preparations fit seamlessly into your daily life, enhancing flavor while providing supportive compounds that improve digestion, immunity, or overall well-being.

By viewing your pantry as a source of nourishment and healing, you connect more deeply with the simple gifts of nature. Choose quality ingredients, store them properly, and pay attention to how you feel after incorporating them into your routine. Over time, you may find yourself reaching for these kitchen remedies as naturally as you reach for your favorite spice-taking a holistic approach that fuses cooking and wellness into a single art.

- Remedy 236: Garlic Honey Infusion
    - Use: Support immunity, soothe mild sore throats
    - Ingredients: 1–2 garlic cloves, enough honey to cover

- How to Prepare: Crush garlic, cover with honey in jar, let infuse a few days, strain
- Tips: Use a spoonful as needed; store in cool place

- Remedy 237: Onion Syrup for Colds
  - Use: Ease mild coughs and congestion
  - Ingredients: 1 small onion sliced, honey or sugar
  - How to Prepare: Layer onion and sweetener, let sit overnight, strain syrup
  - Tips: Mild onion flavor; take by spoonful as needed

- Remedy 238: Cinnamon Spiced Vinegar
  - Use: Add warmth and subtle digestive support to meals
  - Ingredients: Cinnamon stick, apple cider vinegar
  - How to Prepare: Infuse cinnamon in vinegar for 2–4 weeks, strain
  - Tips: Use in dressings, marinades, or dilute in water

- Remedy 239: Clove Infused Oil
  - Use: Mild antiseptic and warming oil for external use

- Ingredients: Whole cloves, carrier oil
- How to Prepare: Infuse cloves in oil for several weeks, strain
- Tips: Use sparingly on skin; test small area first

- **Remedy 240: Ginger-Honey Immunity Paste**
  - Use: Warm body, support immune function
  - Ingredients: 1 tsp grated ginger, 2 tbsp honey
  - How to Prepare: Mix ginger into honey, let infuse
  - Tips: Stir into hot water or tea; store sealed

- **Remedy 241: Rosemary Salt Seasoning**
  - Use: Flavor foods while adding mild circulatory support
  - Ingredients: Dried rosemary, sea salt
  - How to Prepare: Grind rosemary with salt, store in jar
  - Tips: Use on roasted veggies, meats, or soups

- **Remedy 242: Thyme Infused Olive Oil**
  - Use: Culinary oil with gentle antimicrobial support
  - Ingredients: Fresh thyme sprigs, olive oil

- - How to Prepare: Infuse thyme in oil a few weeks, strain
  - Tips: Drizzle on salads or bread; store in dark place
- Remedy 243: Turmeric Golden Paste
  - Use: Anti-inflammatory boost for meals and drinks
  - Ingredients: Ground turmeric, water, pinch black pepper
  - How to Prepare: Simmer turmeric with water to paste, add pepper
  - Tips: Stir into milk, soups, or smoothies
- Remedy 244: Peppermint Sugar Crystals
  - Use: Add fresh aroma and slight digestive support to sweets
  - Ingredients: Fresh peppermint leaves, sugar
  - How to Prepare: Layer leaves with sugar, let dry, sift leaves out
  - Tips: Sprinkle on desserts or fruit
- Remedy 245: Sage Infused Honey
  - Use: Soothing addition to teas, mild antimicrobial support
  - Ingredients: Fresh sage leaves, honey

- How to Prepare: Infuse sage in honey a few weeks, strain

- Tips: Spoon into warm water or tea; store sealed

Chapter 13: Cultural and Traditional Remedies (Remedies 246–250)

Throughout history, communities around the world have relied on local plants and traditional knowledge to maintain health and vitality. These remedies often carry layers of meaning that reflect cultural identity, spiritual practices, and the hard-won wisdom of ancestors. This chapter offers a glimpse into such traditions, reminding us that health is woven into the tapestry of human history.

You will find preparations from diverse backgrounds, each reflecting the flavors, aromas, and healing philosophies of its origin. These remedies highlight common threads such as respect for the earth's adaptability and the principle that nature provides what we need if we learn to see it. They offer an opportunity to connect with cultures beyond our own, expanding our understanding of how people everywhere find comfort and resilience.

Think of these remedies as an invitation to appreciate the universality of healing traditions. Experiment thoughtfully with new tastes, approach the unknown with curiosity, and carry forward the common human quest for wellness. In doing so, you will honor the lineage of knowledge that transcends borders and centuries, uniting us in our common pursuit of health, harmony, and a meaningful life.

- Remedy 246: Ayurvedic Golden Milk (Turmeric)
    - Use: Warm, soothing drink promoting relaxation and gentle anti-inflammatory effect

- Ingredients: 1 tsp turmeric paste, 1 cup warm milk, pinch cinnamon
- How to Prepare: Stir turmeric paste into warm milk, add cinnamon
- Tips: Enjoy before bed; add honey for sweetness

- Remedy 247: TCM Astragalus Immune Broth
  - Use: Support vitality and immune balance in the traditional Chinese method
  - Ingredients: A few slices astragalus root, broth or water
  - How to Prepare: Simmer root in broth, strain, sip warm
  - Tips: Mild, earthy taste; add to soups for daily nourishment

- Remedy 248: European Elderflower Cordial
  - Use: Refreshing beverage supporting mild immunity and relaxation
  - Ingredients: Elderflowers, sugar, lemon, water
  - How to Prepare: Infuse flowers in sugar water with lemon, strain
  - Tips: Dilute with still or sparkling water; store in fridge

- Remedy 249: Indigenous Sage Smoke Cleansing

- Use: Purify space, encourage calm, honor traditional practices
- Ingredients: Dried sage bundle
- How to Prepare: Light sage bundle, blow out flame, waft smoke gently
- Tips: Use respectfully; ensure proper ventilation

- Remedy 250: Mediterranean Rosemary-Garlic Tonic
  - Use: Support circulation, digestion, and overall well-being
  - Ingredients: A sprig rosemary, 1 clove garlic, 1 cup hot water
  - How to Prepare: Steep rosemary and crushed garlic 10 minutes, strain
  - Tips: Strong flavor; add lemon or honey for balance.

Chapter 14: Safety Guidelines and When to Seek Professional Advice (Contraindications, Pediatric Use, Pregnancy Precautions, Medication Interactions)

When working with herbal remedies, it is important to understand not only their potential benefits, but also the limitations and cautions associated with their use. Herbs come from nature, which can be comforting, but this fact alone does not guarantee that every plant is safe for every individual at all times. Just as you would exercise caution and seek professional advice before taking a new pharmaceutical medication or dietary supplement, you should approach herbal preparations with a balanced perspective that respects both their healing potential and their limitations. By doing so, you will help ensure that your journey into herbalism remains positive, beneficial, and free of unnecessary complications. This chapter is intended to guide you through the complex area of herbal safety by examining issues such as contraindications, pediatric considerations, pregnancy precautions, and interactions with commonly prescribed medications.

One of the most important principles to keep in mind is that individuals are unique and respond differently to herbal remedies. Factors such as age, weight, current health status, and genetic predisposition can all influence how you respond to certain herbs. What may be soothing and restorative for one person may be ineffective or even irritating for another. Begin your exploration of herbal remedies with gentle, well-known herbs that have a long history of use and few reported adverse effects. Over time, as you gain confidence, you can gradually introduce new preparations while paying attention to the signals your body is sending you. If you notice any unusual symptoms or discomfort, take a step back, reassess, and, if necessary, seek the advice of a knowledgeable professional.

Contraindications refer to conditions or circumstances in which a particular herb should not be used or should be used only under strict supervision. Some herbs may increase blood pressure, stimulate uterine contractions, or interfere with blood clotting. Others may cause sensitivity in people with autoimmune disorders or allergies. Understanding these contraindications is critical before incorporating any new herb into your self-care routine. If you are unsure, consult a licensed herbalist, naturopathic physician, or other qualified healthcare provider who is knowledgeable about both conventional medicine and traditional herbal practices. They can help you determine whether a particular herb is appropriate for your personal health goals and conditions.

Pediatric use of herbal remedies requires additional caution. Children have developing immune systems and metabolisms that may not process herbs in the same way as adults. In addition, their smaller body size means that dosages intended for adults may be excessive. When preparing remedies for children, choose mild herbs with a strong safety record. Always start with a small amount and watch for any reactions. Teas and syrups are often gentler forms of administration for young children because they allow for easy dilution and pleasant flavors. Remember that children may be more sensitive to bitterness, strong scents, or certain textures. Keep the lines of communication open as appropriate for their age and let them share how they feel after using a remedy. In all cases of pediatric use, it is wise to consult a pediatrician or qualified pediatric herbalist, especially if the child has a known medical condition or is on medication.

Pregnancy adds another layer of complexity. The body undergoes profound changes during pregnancy, and what was previously safe may now need to be avoided. Some herbs can stimulate uterine contractions or affect hormones in ways that are not appropriate for a pregnant individual. Others may be perfectly safe and even supportive, providing gentle nourishment and comfort during a challenging time. The key is to rely on well-established guidelines and professional advice. Many midwives, herbalists, and integrative health care providers are experienced in selecting herbs that can safely support common pregnancy-related concerns, such as mild nausea, digestive problems, or stress. Always share your herbal plans with a trusted healthcare provider who understands both sides of the coin. If uncertainty persists, err on the side of caution and avoid taking any herb without clear, reliable guidance.

Lactation is similarly sensitive. Just as certain herbs can increase milk flow, others can decrease it or impart an undesirable taste to breast milk. Some may even indirectly affect the nursing infant. Approach this phase with caution and professional advice. Choose simple, gentle remedies that are commonly recommended and well-documented for nursing mothers. When trying a new herb, pay close attention to your own well-being as well as any subtle changes in your infant, such as fussiness, altered sleep patterns, or digestive discomfort. This careful observation can alert you early on if a particular herb is not being well tolerated.

Drug interactions are another important aspect of herbal safety. Many people today rely on prescription medications to manage chronic conditions, stabilize moods, or control blood pressure, cholesterol, and other health parameters. Certain herbs can interact with these medications in unintended ways. For example, St. John's wort, known for its mood-lifting properties, can speed up the metabolism of some drugs, making them less effective. Licorice root can increase blood pressure, which could be problematic if combined with medications used for high blood pressure. It is important to tell your healthcare provider about all the herbal remedies you are taking so they can monitor for potential interactions and adjust prescriptions as needed. This transparency fosters a team-based approach to your health, ensuring that all therapies work in harmony rather than at cross-purposes.

Another consideration is the source and quality of your herbs. Contamination with heavy metals, pesticides, or adulterants can cause unwanted side effects. Always choose reputable suppliers who are transparent about their sourcing and processing methods. Organic certifications and third-party testing can be good indicators of quality. Proper identification is also essential, especially when foraging for wild plants. Mistaking a poisonous lookalike for a beneficial herb can result in serious harm. Consulting field guides or experienced foragers can help prevent tragic mistakes. If uncertainty persists, rely on dried herbs from trusted herbal shops rather than harvesting your own.

When evaluating the safety of an herb, look for several reputable sources of information. Peer-reviewed studies, respected herbal textbooks, and experienced herbalists can all provide valuable insight. Remember that just because a remedy is traditional does not guarantee safety for your particular situation. Traditions have evolved over time, and what worked well in one setting or population may not transfer seamlessly to another. Historical records can be a starting point, but modern research offers additional data on efficacy, dosage ranges, and reported side effects. Balancing ancient wisdom with contemporary evidence-based knowledge creates a more reliable foundation for your herbal practice.

Knowing when to seek professional advice is an integral part of responsible herbal use. If you experience severe or persistent symptoms such as severe abdominal pain, difficulty breathing, high fever, confusion, or rapid changes in heart rate, stop using the herb and consult a qualified healthcare provider immediately. Herbs are not a substitute for emergency medical care. If you have a serious health condition such as diabetes, cancer, heart disease, or an autoimmune disorder, approach herbal remedies with caution. Work with an integrative health care provider who can help you safely incorporate herbs as appropriate. If you are planning surgery, inform your medical team about any herbs you are taking, as some may affect bleeding or interact with anesthesia.

It is also wise to consider the psychological aspect of herbal use. Expectations can shape results in subtle ways. Placebo effects are well documented in both conventional and alternative medicine. If you strongly believe in an herb's ability to heal, you may feel better just by taking it, even if the herb itself has a mild effect. Conversely, if you are suspicious or fearful, you may interpret harmless side effects as evidence that the herb is harmful. Maintaining an open but critical mindset will help you navigate these psychological factors. Objectively observe and record your experiences. When in doubt, seek a second opinion from a professional who can provide reassurance or suggest alternatives.

Dosage control is another cornerstone of safety. More is not always better. Some herbs are very potent, and taking them in large amounts can overload the body, leading to toxicity or unwanted side effects. Follow recommended dosages from reputable sources and start at the low end of the range, especially if you are new to a particular herb. Keep track of how it affects you and only increase the dosage if you are sure it is necessary and safe. Remember that herbal remedies often work gradually, so patience is important. Taking large amounts in hopes of a quick fix can backfire.

Sustainability and environmental responsibility are also indirectly linked to safety considerations. By supporting ethical harvesting practices and choosing herbs that are cultivated rather than wild, you help maintain the natural balance of ecosystems. Overharvesting certain wild species can threaten biodiversity and reduce the availability of important medicinal plants for future generations. Ensuring the longevity of these resources allows future herbalists and health seekers to benefit from nature's pharmacy.

Cultural sensitivity and context also play a role in the safe use of herbs. Some herbs may be deeply integrated into certain cultures, with well-established protocols that ensure their safe use. Others may be more experimental or recently incorporated into your own tradition. Learning from cultures that have maintained a long history of safe and effective herbal practice can provide insights into proper dosage preparation and contraindications that may not be well documented in modern literature. However, this cultural exchange should always be approached with respect for the intellectual property traditions and communities that have preserved this knowledge.

As you become more experienced with herbs, you will likely develop an intuitive sense of what feels right for your body. This intuition is valuable, but it should never replace rational judgment and professional input when needed. Health is a dynamic interplay of physical, mental, emotional, and environmental factors. Herbs can support this complexity, but they cannot erase it. Recognize the limits of what herbal remedies can accomplish. They are part of a larger toolkit that includes conventional medicine, nutrition, exercise, stress management, and social support. By weaving these elements together, you create a stronger, healthier foundation for yourself.

In conclusion, safety in herbal practice relies on a combination of careful research, personal mindfulness, professional guidance, and respect for the plants you use. Taking the time to understand contraindications, pediatric considerations, pregnancy precautions, and drug interactions ensures that you are acting responsibly toward yourself, your family, and the herbal community. Do not hesitate to seek help when you need it, and continue to learn as you go. As you gain knowledge and experience, you will gain the confidence to make informed decisions. This empowers you to embrace the profound gifts of nature's pharmacy while safeguarding your well-being and that of the people who rely on you. In doing so, you honor the traditions of herbal healing and preserve them as living treasures that adapt and grow with each generation.

Chapter 15: Preserving Knowledge and Passing It Forward (Keeping an Herbal Journal, Sharing Wisdom, Further Reading and Resources)

Herbal knowledge is not a static set of facts stored in dusty volumes. It is a living tapestry woven from thousands of threads - family traditions, community practices, indigenous wisdom, scientific discoveries, personal anecdotes, and cross-cultural exchanges. Over the centuries, healers, gardeners, midwives, monks, scientists, and everyday people have contributed to its richness. This chapter invites you to step into this tapestry and participate in its ongoing creation. By learning how to preserve your personal experiences, share insights with others, and explore reliable resources, you can help ensure that herbal wisdom continues to thrive in an age when convenience and quick fixes often overshadow time-honored practices.

A fundamental tool for nurturing this heritage is the humble herbal journal. A journal allows you to record your encounters with plants: what remedies you tried, how you prepared them, what symptoms they addressed, and how you felt afterwards. It can be as simple as a notebook or as elaborate as a leather-bound tome filled with illustrations, pressed flowers, and personal reflections. What is important is that you document your learning process. Over time, these records become invaluable guides. They remind you of what worked well, which methods of preparation were most effective, and how particular herbs resonated with your unique body and circumstances. They also help you track subtle changes-whether a particular remedy gradually improved your digestion, or how a blend of calming herbs improved your sleep over several months.

Consistency is important when keeping an herbal journal. Even short notes can be invaluable. Consider including details such as date, time of day, environmental conditions, dosage, and any other therapies you have used. Also document your mood, stress levels, and dietary habits. Often the effects of herbal remedies cannot be completely separated from lifestyle factors. For example, if you notice that an herbal infusion seemed to help your anxiety on a day when you also practiced yoga and took a long walk in the fresh air, you may begin to see patterns. Over time, your journal becomes a map of your healing journey, showing how plants fit into your daily life and personal evolution.

Your journal can also serve as a place for deeper reflection. Herbs are not just chemical compounds; they carry stories, symbolism, and connections to the natural world. Perhaps a sip of chamomile tea reminds you of afternoons in your grandmother's kitchen. Perhaps a lavender bath helps you remember a particular summer field scented with blossoms. By capturing these emotional and sensory responses, you add layers of meaning to your practice. After all, healing is not just about relieving symptoms; it often involves cultivating a sense of connection, purpose, and inner peace. The journal bears witness to these subtle shifts and preserves them for you to revisit when challenges arise or when you need reassurance that growth is possible.

Beyond personal documentation, consider how you might share this knowledge. Teaching others can take many forms. You might start close to home by offering a friend a cup of digestive tea that you have found helpful, explaining how and why it works. Or you could share a simple ointment recipe with a neighbor who has dry skin. Over time, you could lead a small workshop in your community, introducing participants to basic herbal preparations. These small acts of generosity encourage others to explore natural wellness, and you help ensure that this legacy is not lost. Just as you have benefited from the insights of authors, mentors, or elders, you now have the opportunity to become a link in the chain - an integral part of the transmission of knowledge.

Remember that teaching does not require perfection. You do not have to be a master herbalist to share what you have learned so far. Humility goes a long way. Be honest about what you know and what you are still figuring out. Invite others to question, experiment, and refine the knowledge themselves. This openness fosters a sense of community around herbal healing. It reinforces the idea that we are all students, always learning from each other and from the plants themselves. By encouraging dialogue and collaboration, you create a living network rather than a rigid hierarchy.

In today's world, there are many platforms for sharing information. Social media, blogs, online forums, and virtual workshops allow you to connect with people around the world. While the wealth of information available online can be both exciting and overwhelming, it also offers opportunities to build communities of like-minded individuals who support each other's growth. Participate thoughtfully in these spaces. Look for reputable groups or forums moderated by experienced herbalists. Ask thoughtful questions and share your experiences without making claims beyond your expertise. By contributing respectfully, you help maintain the integrity and usefulness of these communities.

Offline, do not underestimate the power of face-to-face connections. Community gardens, herbal study groups, and local health-focused gatherings can be meaningful avenues for interaction. When people come together around a common interest, they bring different backgrounds, skills, and perspectives. Someone may have a family tradition about plants from a region you have never visited. Another person may offer scientific insights from their professional training. These convergences enrich everyone's understanding and ensure that herbal knowledge remains dynamic and inclusive.

As you move beyond your immediate circle, consider making your knowledge more widely available. Writing articles, contributing to newsletters, or even collaborating on a local herbal zine can spread valuable information. You could also donate herbal reference books to your local library or health center, ensuring that curious readers have accessible resources at their fingertips. If you have expertise in a particular area-perhaps you have mastered the art of making herbal syrups or have extensive experience growing medicinal plants in an urban environment-consider creating a small booklet or guide. These tangible contributions can reach people you have never met, planting seeds of inspiration that may bloom long after you have shared the information.

In addition to sharing your own findings, it is wise to continue to learn and expand your horizons. Herbalism is vast, encompassing traditions from every continent and countless cultural contexts. Explore resources that will challenge your assumptions and broaden your perspective. Explore the writings of herbalists who specialize in Traditional Chinese Medicine or Ayurveda. Investigate the herbal practices of indigenous peoples while respecting their intellectual property rights and ensuring that your learning is guided by respect, permission, and cultural sensitivity. In doing so, you acknowledge that no single tradition has all the answers. This humility and curiosity will help you grow as a lifelong student of nature's pharmacy.

In your quest for credible information, be prepared to engage with both historical and modern sources. Ancient texts, ethnobotanical studies, and folklore reveal how our ancestors worked in harmony with the land. They remind us that people survived and thrived long before the advent of modern medicine. At the same time, scientific research and clinical trials provide valuable insights into active ingredients, safety profiles and precise dosages. Balancing these perspectives gives you a well-rounded understanding. It also helps you communicate with a variety of audiences. Someone rooted in tradition may appreciate references to cultural practices, while a scientifically inclined friend may find it reassuring that modern studies support the efficacy of a particular herb.

When evaluating sources, consider their credibility, transparency, and context. Reputable authors and researchers often cite their sources, acknowledge limitations, and encourage critical thinking. Be wary of sources that make grandiose claims without evidence. Hyperbole and miracle cures are red flags that can lead to disappointment or even harm. As you refine your critical eye, you will become better at sifting through the noise and finding gems of wisdom in a sea of misinformation.

Your journey into herbalism can be enhanced by seeking out structured learning opportunities. Workshops, courses, apprenticeships, or mentorships with experienced herbalists provide hands-on training, immediate feedback, and opportunities for in-depth exploration. These learning experiences can deepen your confidence and refine your skills. They also put you in a supportive network, making it easier to find reliable guidance when challenges arise.

While preserving and passing on knowledge is crucial, remember that this tradition is not about creating rigid dogma. Herbalism thrives on adaptation and innovation. As climates change, plants migrate, and societal needs evolve, so do the remedies and approaches we use. Keeping an open mind means recognizing that some practices may need to be updated. For example, if a particular plant becomes endangered due to habitat loss, responsible herbalists seek sustainable alternatives. If modern research reveals a previously unknown interaction or contraindication, informed practitioners adjust their recommendations accordingly. This adaptability ensures that knowledge remains relevant and effective for future generations.

The interplay between oral traditions and written records is another point to consider. Much herbal knowledge has historically been passed down through storytelling and apprenticeship, with grandparents teaching grandchildren and community elders guiding aspiring healers. Written texts and modern recordings support this chain of transmission, ensuring that the teachings survive beyond an individual's lifetime. Your herbal journal and your efforts to share knowledge contribute to this continuum, combining ancient ways of learning with today's technological resources.

Preserving knowledge also means respecting cultural boundaries and intellectual property. Many indigenous communities hold sacred knowledge about local plants, their uses, and their spiritual significance. Approaching these traditions with humility, seeking permission, and acknowledging the source of the wisdom are critical steps. Extracting knowledge without giving credit or reciprocity can perpetuate colonial attitudes and harm the communities that have safeguarded this information for generations. Ethical engagement ensures that herbalism remains a force for healing and unity rather than a tool for exploitation.

Sharing knowledge is not just about information; it is also about inspiration. When you share your experiences, you spark curiosity in others. Perhaps a friend who never considered nature's role in healing will pay closer attention to the plants in her backyard. Or maybe a family member struggling with stress will find solace in a soothing tea you recommended. Over time, this awareness can inspire people to become better stewards of the environment, recognizing that the health of the planet and human health are inextricably linked. In this sense, every piece of knowledge you share has the potential to shape how people interact with the natural world.

To help you continue to grow, this book includes references and resources in the appendices. There you will find suggestions for further reading, reliable suppliers, and tools to enhance your herb identification skills. As you explore these resources, you will deepen your confidence and expand your toolkit. Think of each reference as a stepping stone on a path that can take you through botanical gardens, historical archives, molecular research labs, and traditional kitchens around the world.

If you feel called to specialize in an area-such as women's health, respiratory disease, or culinary herbs-additional research and collaboration with experts can help you build a solid knowledge base. Over time, you could become a local go-to person for that specialty, helping others overcome specific challenges with informed suggestions. This does not mean memorizing every detail. Instead, it means knowing where to look when a question arises. Your journal, your library, and your community all serve as living references.

As you gather and share knowledge, remember to celebrate successes and acknowledge stumbling blocks. Not every tool will produce the desired result. Some experiments may fail, or you may find conflicting information that requires deeper investigation. These moments are not defeats. They are opportunities to learn, to refine your understanding, and to sharpen your discernment. The practice of herbalism is a cycle of exploration, feedback, and growth-much like the cycles of the seasons that nourish the plants we rely on.

In addition to sharing on a personal and community level, consider ways you can contribute to the broader field. This could include writing letters to the editors of herbal journals, participating in citizen science projects that track plant populations, or collaborating with researchers who need data on traditional uses of particular herbs. In this way, you become an active participant in the ongoing development of herbal knowledge. Your observations may one day inform larger studies, shape best practices, or guide policy decisions related to herbal medicines.

Another valuable dimension is mentorship. As you gain experience, you may find yourself mentoring someone who is just starting out. This could be as simple as suggesting a beginner-friendly herb or demonstrating how to make a basic tincture. Acting as a mentor helps to solidify your own understanding. Teaching someone else often clarifies what you know well and what you need to revisit. It is also deeply rewarding to see the spark of curiosity ignited in another person.

As you continue to record, share, and seek knowledge, try to maintain a balance. Do not let the quest for information overshadow the simple pleasure of connecting with plants and enjoying their gentle gifts. Sometimes it is enough to savor the aroma of a steaming cup of tea, feel the soothing warmth of an ointment on your skin, or admire the grace of a wild flower swaying in the breeze. Herbalism is both a science and an art. While knowledge is its backbone, intuition and appreciation are its heart and soul.

In the great tapestry of human history, countless individuals have contributed threads of knowledge about herbal healing. By preserving your own insights, sharing them with others, and continually expanding your understanding, you ensure that this tapestry remains vibrant, colorful, and ever-growing. You play a vital role in ensuring that future generations will have access to these time-tested remedies, these gentle allies from the plant kingdom, and the wisdom woven through them.

As you put these pages into practice, remember that you are not walking this path alone. You are walking alongside countless others who have come before you, those who are walking with you now, and those who will follow. By treasuring what you learn, sharing what you know, and always striving to grow, you help ensure that herbal knowledge will endure and provide comfort, healing, and inspiration for generations to come.

Conclusion.

As you turn the final pages of this book and reflect on its contents, remember that you have tapped into a legacy that goes far beyond these words. The remedies gathered here, drawn from traditions carefully preserved and renewed, represent more than a collection of useful recipes. They symbolize a way back to an understanding that true wellness often lies not in complexity or costly intervention, but in the simple gifts of nature, lovingly prepared and thoughtfully applied. By embracing these ancient methods, you become part of a continuum that honors those who have gone before and lights the way for those who will follow.

The journey you have taken through these pages has provided a framework for seeing herbs not as distant curiosities, but as living allies present in your kitchen, your garden, and the landscapes you explore. As you blend tinctures, brew infusions, and prepare soothing balms, you weave threads of tradition into your modern life. Each cup of tea sipped with intention and each salve gently massaged into the skin reminds you that health can be cultivated through mindful awareness, compassionate self-care, and respect for the harmony between humanity and the plant world.

May this knowledge inspire you to continue to learn, share, and grow in your understanding of nature's pharmacy. Keep exploring new herbs, refining your preparations, and documenting your experiences so that you can pass on this wisdom. In doing so, you ensure that what may have been lost remains vibrant and alive, available to anyone willing to listen, observe, and learn. Let your herbal practice be a source of comfort, resilience, and hope, and let the gifts of Barbara O'Neill's forgotten apothecary guide you toward a life more deeply rooted in connection and well-being.

Margaret Willowbrook

LAST WORD.

Before you set this book aside, pause to recognize the enduring wisdom it carries. The remedies and traditions within these pages reflect more than individual recipes—they represent a timeless approach to wellness that draws on nature's quiet generosity. By choosing to engage with these methods, you are stepping into a lineage that stretches back through countless generations, each one passing forward insight, experience, and trust in the healing power of simple, well-chosen herbs.

As you continue to stir tinctures, steep infusions, and craft salves, remember that you are not walking this path alone. The plants you tend and the remedies you create weave your personal story into a much larger tapestry. With each careful preparation, each sip savored, and each moment spent in observation of the natural world, you become both student and teacher, both recipient and steward of this living tradition.

May your connection to these practices remain fluid and evolving. Keep exploring new techniques, refining your skills, and noting your observations in a journal, so that you, too, can add a thread of understanding for those who will learn from you someday. In this way, the legacy of Barbara O'Neill's forgotten apothecary continues to flourish, ensuring that nature's gifts and the knowledge they inspire remain accessible, meaningful, and alive for generations to come.

GLOSSARY OF HERBAL TERMS

Adaptogen: A substance believed to help the body adapt to stress and maintain homeostasis by supporting normal metabolic processes and reducing fatigue.

Alterative: An herb that gradually restores proper function to the body and increases overall health and vitality by improving elimination and metabolism.

Analgesic: An herb that helps reduce or relieve pain without causing loss of consciousness.

Anodyne: Similar to analgesic, a substance that soothes pain and eases discomfort, often applied topically.

Anthraquinone Glycoside: A type of compound commonly found in certain laxative herbs; these compounds influence bowel movements and intestinal contractions.

Anti-inflammatory: An herb or compound that helps reduce inflammation in the body, often easing pain and swelling.

Antimicrobial: A substance that helps kill or inhibit the growth of microorganisms such as bacteria, viruses, or fungi.

Antioxidant: A compound that helps protect cells from damage caused by free radicals, supporting overall health and longevity.

Aromatic: Herbs rich in volatile oils, producing a strong fragrance that can improve flavor, aid digestion, and sometimes support respiratory health.

Astringent: A substance that causes tissues to tighten, contract, and become less permeable, often used to reduce bleeding, secretions, or inflammation.

Bitter: A flavor profile indicating the presence of compounds that can stimulate digestion by increasing saliva, stomach acid, and bile flow.

Carminative: An herb that helps ease gas and bloating by relaxing intestinal muscles and promoting the release of trapped gas.

Cholagogue: A substance that stimulates the production and release of bile from the liver and gallbladder, aiding digestion and fat metabolism.

Circulatory Stimulant: An herb that helps improve blood flow, warming the body and supporting healthy circulation.

Decoction: A method of herbal preparation that involves simmering tougher plant materials like roots and bark in water to extract their active constituents.

Demulcent: An herb that soothes and protects irritated or inflamed tissues, often high in mucilage and beneficial for respiratory or digestive tracts.

Diaphoretic: A substance that induces sweating, often used to help the body regulate temperature and eliminate toxins through the skin.

Diuretic: An herb that increases urine production, helping the body remove excess fluid and support kidney function.

Emetic: A substance that induces vomiting, sometimes used to expel toxins from the stomach.

Emmenagogue: An herb that helps stimulate or regulate menstrual flow and may support overall reproductive health.

Essential Oil: Highly concentrated volatile oil extracted from aromatic plants, containing the plant's characteristic fragrance and many active compounds.

Febrifuge: A remedy that helps reduce or prevent fever by cooling the body and supporting the immune response.

Flavonoid: A class of plant compounds with antioxidant properties, often contributing to the color and health benefits of many herbs.

Galactagogue: An herb that can support or increase the production of breast milk in nursing mothers.

Hepatoprotective: A substance that helps protect liver cells from damage, supporting healthy liver function.

Infusion: A method of extracting an herb's active constituents by steeping delicate plant parts like leaves or flowers in hot water.

Latex: A milky fluid found in some plants that can contain medicinal compounds; often associated with herbs that have laxative or soothing properties.

Laxative: An herb that stimulates or facilitates bowel movements, easing constipation and promoting regularity.

Maceration: A technique of soaking herbs in a solvent (often cold water or alcohol) for a period of time to extract their active constituents.

Menorrhagia: Excessive or prolonged menstrual bleeding; some herbs may be used to help reduce heavy flow.

Menstruum: The solvent used to extract an herb's active compounds, often alcohol, water, glycerin, or vinegar.

Nervine: An herb that acts on the nervous system, calming the nerves, easing anxiety, or restoring balance and vitality.

Oxymel: A traditional preparation made by combining honey and vinegar, often used as a base for herbal remedies that support respiratory health.

Pectoral: An herb that supports the health of the lungs and respiratory system, often soothing coughs or easing congestion.

Percolation: A method of extracting herbal constituents by passing a solvent slowly through a bed of coarsely ground plant material.

Phytochemical: A naturally occurring plant compound that can have beneficial effects on human health.

Poultice: A soft, moist preparation of herbs applied topically to soothe inflammation, draw out impurities, or promote healing.

Relaxant: An herb that helps calm tense muscles and relieve nervous tension, promoting relaxation and ease.

Resins: Sticky plant secretions that contain aromatic and medicinal compounds, often used in tinctures or topical preparations.

Rubefacient: A substance that increases blood flow to the skin's surface, producing a warming sensation and sometimes relieving muscle aches.

Saponin: A plant compound that creates a soap-like foam in water and may help the body absorb certain nutrients, sometimes influencing metabolism or cholesterol.

Sedative: An herb that helps calm the nervous system, encouraging rest, sleep, and a reduction in anxious feelings.

Simple: A preparation or remedy using only one herb, allowing you to understand its specific effects and qualities.

Solvent: The medium used to extract compounds from plant materials, such as water, alcohol, glycerin, or vinegar.

Spasmolytic: An herb that helps reduce or prevent muscle spasms, easing cramps and tension.

Styptic: A substance that helps stop bleeding by causing blood vessels to contract and tissues to tighten.

Tannin: A plant compound known for its astringent properties, often found in bark and leaves, useful for toning tissues and reducing inflammation.

Tincture: A concentrated herbal extract made by soaking plant material in alcohol or a mixture of alcohol and water, preserving compounds for long-term use.

Tonifying: An action of gently strengthening and supporting specific organs or systems over time without overstimulation.

Tonic: An herb that supports overall wellness and vitality, often working slowly and steadily to improve bodily functions.

Vulnerary: A substance that aids in wound healing, helping tissues regenerate and reducing infection risk.

Conversion Tables.

Use these tables to convert measurements commonly found in herbal recipes. Adjusting between metric and imperial units ensures that you can follow any recipe accurately, regardless of its origin.

Volume Conversions

1 teaspoon (tsp) ≈ 5 milliliters (mL)
1 tablespoon (tbsp) ≈ 15 milliliters (mL)
1 fluid ounce (fl oz) ≈ 30 milliliters (mL)
1 cup ≈ 240 milliliters (mL)
1 pint ≈ 480 milliliters (mL)
1 quart ≈ 960 milliliters (mL)
1 gallon ≈ 3840 milliliters (mL) or 3.84 liters (L)

Weight Conversions

1 ounce (oz) ≈ 28 grams (g)
1 pound (lb) ≈ 454 grams (g) or approximately 0.45 kilograms (kg)
For small herbal measures: 1 gram ≈ 0.035 ounces

Length Conversions

1 inch ≈ 2.54 centimeters (cm)
1 foot (12 inches) ≈ 30.48 centimeters (cm)
1 meter ≈ 39.37 inches

Approximate Herbal Measures

A handful of fresh herbs ≈ 1/4 to 1/2 cup loosely packed leaves
A pinch ≈ a small amount easily taken between thumb and forefinger, often about 1/8 teaspoon.

Tips for Accuracy

Use a kitchen scale for precise weight measurements, especially when working with dried herbs.

Use graduated measuring spoons and cups for liquids and powdered herbs.

When in doubt, start with the lower recommended measurement and adjust gradually to achieve desired strength or consistency.

REFERENCES

1. Pursell, JJ. THE HERBAL APOTHECARY: 100 MEDICINAL HERBS AND HOW TO USE THEM. Timber Press, 2015.

2. Green, James. THE HERBAL MEDICINE-MAKER'S HANDBOOK: A HOME MANUAL. Crossing Press, 2000.

3. Cech, Richo. MAKING PLANT MEDICINE. Horizon Herbs, 2000.

4. McIntyre, Anne. THE COMPLETE HERBAL TUTOR: THE DEFINITIVE GUIDE TO THE PRINCIPLES AND PRACTICES OF HERBAL MEDICINE. Gaia Books, 2010.

5. Gladstar, Rosemary. ROSEMARY GLADSTAR'S MEDICINAL HERBS: A BEGINNER'S GUIDE. Storey Publishing, 2012.

6. Kloss, Jethro. BACK TO EDEN: THE CLASSIC GUIDE TO HERBAL MEDICINE, NATURAL FOODS, AND HOME REMEDIES SINCE 1939. Lotus Press, 1939.

7. Levy, Juliette de Bairacli. COMMON HERBS FOR NATURAL HEALTH. Ash Tree Publishing, 1974.

8. Fischer-Rizzi, Susanne. COMPLETE EARTH MEDICINE HANDBOOK: NATURAL HEALING WITH HERBS, ESSENTIAL OILS, AND FLOWER ESSENCES. Sterling Publishing, 1996.

9. Hernandez, Mimi Prunella. HERBAL: 100 HERBS FROM THE WORLD'S HEALING TRADITIONS. Ivy Press, 2021.

10. Tierra, Michael. THE WAY OF HERBS. Pocket Books, 1998.

11. De la Forêt, Rosalee. ALCHEMY OF HERBS: TRANSFORM EVERYDAY INGREDIENTS INTO FOODS AND REMEDIES THAT HEAL. Hay House Inc., 2017.

12. Gladstar, Rosemary. HERBAL RECIPES FOR VIBRANT HEALTH. Storey Publishing, 2008.

13. Books, seminars, and lectures by Barbara O'Neill, a leading natural health educator and naturopath.

BONUS PAGE: VIDEO SHORT TUTORIALS BY BARBARA O'NEILL

Thank you for joining us on this journey through the world of herbal healing and natural medicine. To enrich your learning experience, we're thrilled to offer you exclusive access to a collection of video short tutorials featuring Barbara O'Neil. These tutorials, extracted directly from her lectures, provide practical, visual guidance on implementing the natural health practices discussed in this book.

By subscribing, you'll not only gain instant access to our current video library but also be updated with new videos as we continue to add to our collection. This is a fantastic way to stay connected with the latest in herbal healing and natural medicine, ensuring you're always equipped with the knowledge to support your wellness journey.

How to Access:

Simply scan the QR code below or follow the provided link to subscribe and unlock your access. This is our way of saying thank you and enhancing your journey toward holistic health with the invaluable wisdom of Barbara O'Neill.

@INFINITEWELLNESSWAVE

https://www.instagram.com/infinitewellnesswave

As new tutorials become available, you'll be the first to know, allowing you to continuously expand your understanding and application of natural health principles.

We hope these video tutorials serve as a valuable resource in your quest for wellness, bringing the teachings of Barbara O'Neill to life in a new and engaging way. Your feedback and suggestions are always welcome as we grow this library together.